DATABOOK ON GERIATRICS

G. S. RAI MD, MSc, MRCP

V. PEARCE MB, BSc, MRCP

Senior Registrars
Department of Geriatrics
Cambridgeshire Area Health Authority

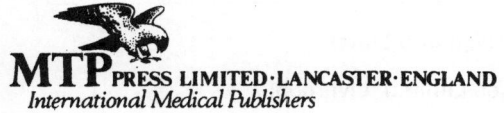
MTP PRESS LIMITED·LANCASTER·ENGLAND
International Medical Publishers

Published by

MTP Press Limited
Falcon House
Lancaster, England.

First published 1980

British Library Cataloguing in Publication Data

Rai, G S
   Databook on geriatrics.
   1.   Geriatrics
   I.   Title   II. Pearce, V
   618.9'7   RC952

   ISBN-13:978-94-009-8702-9   e-ISBN-13:978-94-009-8700-5
   DOI: 10.1007/978-94-009-8700-5

REDWOOD BURN LIMITED, Trowbridge and Esher

Phototypesetting by Swiftpages Limited, Liverpool.

Preface

The aim of these short notes is to provide the newcomer to the speciality of geriatrics with a wide though not exhaustive differential diagnosis of most of the commonly encountered symptoms in the elderly, and to draw particular attention to the common and important disorders. The common causes of symptoms and the common diseases as well as certain features which have special importance to the medicine of the elderly are emphasized.

A final section on investigations (with short notes) which one may employ in the practice of geriatric medicine is included along with an appendix of normal values for the elderly.

In our view this book does not show how geriatric medicine is practised but it does provide an outline of clinical aspects of medicine (geriatrics), knowledge of which is essential to the practice of geriatrics.

G.S.R.
V.P.

Foreword

I take the view that if vitality is reduced to the extent that it interferes with life as the old person would wish to live it, then a proper medical assessment should be made as part of the overall appraisal of that person's problems. The provision of a home help or the meals on wheels service cannot be expected to revitalize the person suffering from hypothroidism or pernicious anaemia! In the event both medical treatment and social support may be needed and to provide one without the other would be half measures.

The medical content of ill-health in old people is considerable in both its extent and complexity – this explains the heavy utilization of medical services by the age group as a whole and by the very old in particular. Much disease in the elderly (as in other age groups) has a large social and a variable psychiatric component, but until the dawn of the era of the universally healthy life style doctors will have plenty of medical work to keep them busy. Obviously, the medical aspects of illness in old age are not the prerogative of the geriatrician. Nevertheless, if he offers an open access service most of the very old people coming to hospital with medical problems will be referred to him, whereas the majority of the younger elderly may continue to be referred to the general medical department. In Cambridge the mean age of admission to the geriatric department is around 80 years, which is almost two decades higher than the mean age of admission to a general medical ward. These very old people present special problems of medical diagnosis and treatment and their illnesses represent a formidable diagnostic and therapeutic challenge which is the very essence of geriatrics.

Geriatrics is not all 'strokes, arthritis, and senile dementia' any more than general medicine is all 'drug overdoses, coronaries and anxiety neurosis'. Admittedly the casual observer might be forgiven for thinking otherwise! Of course common illnesses occur commonly and the good doctor is well aware of the fact. However, he is also aware that less common diseases do occur and that even the common diseases can masquerade to the extent they are virtually unrecognizable. Furthermore, the cases sent in to hospital are not just a random selection of illness in old age but are selected in such a way that the acute geriatric ward always has a goodly selection of the bizarre to tax the imagination and skill of the medical staff. Geriatric medicine is deep as well as wide but the depths are not always well explored except in a few areas.

I hope that *Databook on Geriatrics,* written by two young clinicians who grapple daily with the wide range of illness in the elderly, will be helpful to others working in this field. The simple tabular presentation provides not only a guide for the junior doctor and an *aide-mémoire* for his senior, but also a splendid set of notes for revision just prior to the examinations in medicine at MB and MRCP level.

WILLIAM DAVISON

Senior Physician,
Department of Geriatric Medicine,
Chesterton Hospital,
Cambridge.

Contents

Contents

Introduction

Geriatric Medicine is concerned with the physically sick or disabled elderly, and may be defined as that part of general medicine concerned with the preventive, social, diagnostic and remedial aspects of disease in old age.

Special emphasis is placed on the social background of each patient in view of its implications for their management. Geriatrics is also concerned with research into all facets of the ageing process and care of the elderly.

The clinical practice of modern geriatrics has been found to be most successfully based on a multidisciplinary approach. The multidisciplinary team (Diagram A) of doctors, nurses, remedial therapists and social workers relies heavily, however, on the active involvement of volunteer workers as well as the patient's relatives and friends. All these individuals co-ordinate their respective abilities for the patient's benefit.

One or other of these individuals may play a more prominent part in one aspect of a patient's management; but as in all medical disciplines, appropriate management depends on an accurate and complete diagnosis. Whilst, in geriatric medicine, a purely pathological diagnosis will be incomplete in the absence of a functional and social assessment, it remains the cornerstone of correct management.

For the doctor to work in the department of geriatrics and to lead the team it is necessary for him to be familiar with the diseases of the elderly and how their presentation, course and management differs from that in younger patients, as well as with the working of the multidisciplinary team. The former can to a certain extent be learnt from books but it, like the latter, is mostly acquired by experience of working in the department of geriatrics.

The Multidisciplinary Team

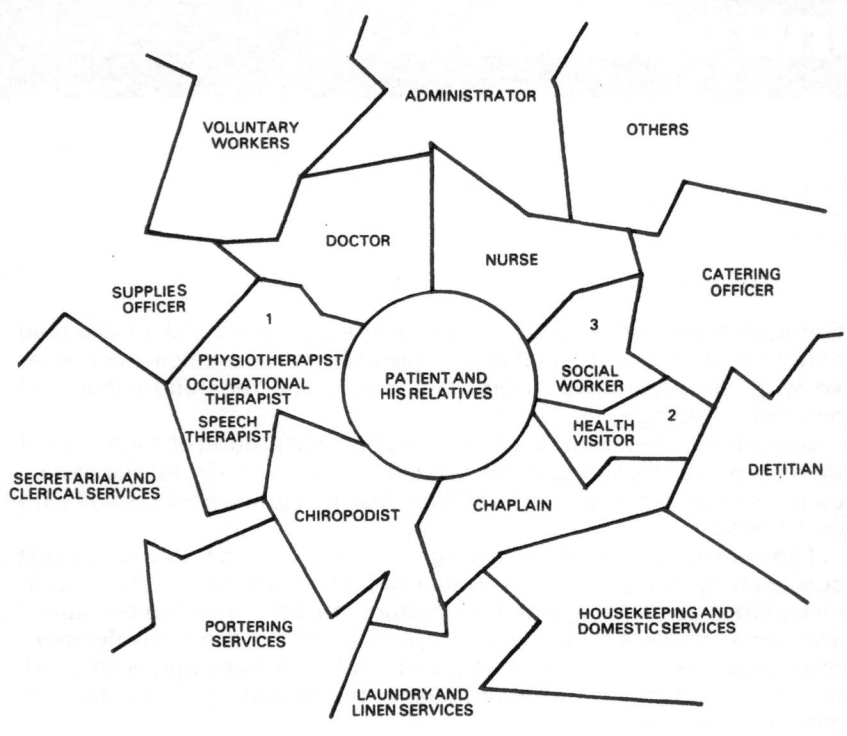

Figure A shows the number of people who might be involved in the multidisciplinary team in the hospital. The diagram with slight modifications is printed from the booklet Improving Geriatric Care in Hospitals *with the kind permission of the Royal College of Nursing.*

[1]Physiotherapist/occupational therapist/speech therapist
    provide rehabilitation and treatment
    assess patient before discharge e.g. ADL (activities of daily living)
    perform home visit to recommend correctable environmental factors prior to discharge
    provide therapy at home in some cases

[2]Health Visitor (geriatric liaison)

    a qualified nurse with a special training in health visiting

    main role is to visit and assess patients at home pre-admission and post-discharge and in hospital prior to discharge.

    pre-admission – to assess the illness and social set up and thus help with early treatment and prevention

    post-discharge – to see that patient is coping without any problems

    pre-discharge – to see patients and relatives to assess their needs before the discharge

[3]Social Worker

    work overlaps somewhat with the health visitor

    provides link between doctor and patient, patient and relatives, doctor and relatives, doctor and social services and patient and social services to achieve best care for the patient (by acting in an advisory role to the multidisciplinary team)

    provides social investigation pre-admission and on out-patients to help with their future care planning

Functions of the Department of Geriatric Medicine

(1) To establish a complete diagnosis in physical, functional and social terms

(2) To correct those disorders amenable to treatment

(3) To rehabilitate and return the patient to the community whenever possible

(4) To identify and correct those factors which may produce disease, preferably before disability has occurred

(5) To maintain as high a level of independence as possible with supports which may range from simple mechanical aids (e.g. commode, walking frame etc.) to more active support such as meals on wheels, home help, district nurse, day centre[i], day hospital[ii] etc.

    When a level of independence cannot be maintained which will allow the patient to remain permanently at home, then assessment for suitability of the patient for intermittent or permanent admission to LARC (local authority residential care) or hospital is carried out. Admission to LARC is arranged with close liaison with the local social services department

3

(6) To operate an intermittent or holiday admissions policy for heavily dependent patients whose relatives are prepared to share the burden of their care. This enables the patient to spend much of his remaining life in his own home surroundings and at the same time gives the family a much deserved break. In addition it temporarily averts the undesirable alternative of permanent hospital care

(7) To provide a continuing care bed in hospital if all supports fail and the patient needs constant nursing care. In the hospital the patient is allowed to live as normal a life as possible within the confines of the hospital

(8) To provide terminal care

[i] day centre
    run by local authority
    provides social contact, food and recreation for independent elderly

[ii] day hospital
    important part of Geriatric department
    provides in-patient facilities on outpatient basis
    main functions
        to continue therapy where necessary once patient has been discharged
        to provide facilities for investigation and to start and continue therapy to patients seen in the OPD and thus prevent admission to hospital
        to provide social contact for patient and relief for relatives during day-time and thus again prevent admission to hospital

Common symptoms

Abdominal Pain

Oesophagus
   oesophagitis
   achalasia
   diffuse spasm

Stomach
   peptic ulceration
   gastric carcinoma
   perforation
   gastritis
   gastric volvulus
   incarcerated hiatus hernia

Small intestine
   ischaemia-intestinal angina
   duodenal diverticulum
   Meckel's diverticulum
   enteritis
   obstruction
   incarceration or strangulation in a hernial orifice

Appendix
   appendicitis

Colon
   diverticular disease
   constipation
   colonic carcinoma
   sigmoid volvulus
   solitary ulcer of caecum
   ischaemic colitis
   pseudomembranous colitis
   spastic colon (irritable bowel)

Other abdominal organs
   liver – hepatitis, primary hepatoma, **liver metastases,** abscess, congestion
   gall bladder and biliary tree – **cholecystitis, cholangitis,** carcinoma of bile duct, carcinoma of gall bladder
   pancreas – **pancreatitis, pancreatic carcinoma**
   spleen – splenic infarct
   kidneys and bladder – renal calculus, **urinary tract infection, renal carcinoma,** bladder papilloma, **urinary retention** etc.
   aorta – leaking aneurysm, dissecting aneurysm

Thoracic
  myocardial infarction
  pneumonia

Metabolic
  hypercalcaemia
  diabetic ketoacidosis – rare

Miscellaneous
  herpes zoster
  radicular pain

Abdominal Swelling

Gaseous
- **constipation**
- **megacolon (idiopathic)**
- intestinal obstruction
- **sigmoid volvulus**
- ileus
- **gastric dilatation** particularly in hypothermia and ketoacidosis

Fluid
- ascites – **neoplastic** – most common
  - secondary to
  - hepatic disease
  - renal disease (nephrotic syndrome – although rare it does occur in the elderly)
  - cardiac disease – constrictive pericarditis
    - constrictive pericarditis
    - congestive heart failure
  - portal or hepatic vein occlusion
  - chronic pancreatitis
  - myxoedema

Organomegaly
- **hepatomegaly**
- splenomegaly
- renal enlargement
- **full bladder**
- **ovarian cyst or tumour**
- fibroids

Miscellaneous
- pancreatic pseudocyst

Chest Pain

Cardiac
> **myocardial infarction**
> **pericarditis** (idiopathic, Dressler's syndrome etc.)
> aortic dissecting aneurysm

Respiratory
> **pulmonary infarction**
> **pleurisy**
> mesothelioma
> **bronchogenic carcinoma**
> pneumothorax

Musculoskeletal
> **fractured ribs**
> **intervertebral disc herniation**
> arthritis of costo-vertebral joints (Tietze's disease)
> myositis
> **metastatic involvement of ribs or sternum**
> Bornholm's disease (NB. chest pain can be absent)

Gastrointestinal
> **hiatus hernia with oesophageal reflux**
> **diffuse spasm (achalasia)**
> **gaseous distension of stomach**
> **peptic ulceration**
> **chronic cholecystitis**

Miscellaneous
> psychogenic
> **osteomalacia**
> **herpes zoster involving thoracic nerve roots**

Cough

Larynx
> **laryngitis**
> **polyp**
> **carcinoma**

chronic bronchitis; asthma
carcinoma – primary bronchogenic or secondary in the lung
pneumonia
TB
pulmonary oedema
subphrenic abscess
mediastinal lymph node enlargement
aortic aneurysm
psychogenic

Recurrent aspiration
> achalasia of cardia
> **neurogenic dysphagia**

Deafness

External auditory meatus
- **wax**
- polyp
- foreign body

perforation of tympanic membrane
otitis media
carcinoma of middle ear
otosclerosis
Ménière's syndrome
fracture through temporal bone

Viral infections
- herpes zoster causing perceptive deafness
- mumps

VIII Nerve Tumour – acoustic neuroma

Drugs
- quinine
- streptomycin
- neomycin
- ethacrynic acid
- frusemide transiently

Presbyacusis
- commonest cause in the elderly
- complex pathophysiology – sensory neural hearing loss of between 10–60 dB

Diarrhoea

Gastric causes
    following gastrectomy or vagotomy

Small intestinal causes
    malabsorption – see p. 126
    change in bowel flora
    Crohn's disease
    ileal resection

Colonic causes
    constipation with overflow
    diverticular disease
    ischaemic colitis
    ulcerative colitis
    pseudomembranous colitis
    villous adenoma
    colonic carcinoma
    infective diarrhoea – Salmonella, Shigella etc.
    ileo-colic fistula

Metabolic
    diabetes mellitus
    thyrotoxicosis
    uraemia
    carcinoid syndrome
    medullary carcinoma of thyroid
    hypoparathyroidism
    Zollinger–Ellison syndrome

Drugs
    antibiotics
    purgatives (abuse)
    cholestyramine

Autonomic neuropathy
    primary
    secondary – diabetes mellitus

Diplopia

Cataract

Orbital lesions displacing the eye
    neoplasm
    abscess
    haemorrhage
    pseudotumour

Ocular palsies
    meningitis
    raised intracranial pressure
    intracranial tumour
    intracranial aneurysm
    cerebrovascular accident
    fracture of skull
    diabetes mellitus
    tabes dorsalis
    Wernicke's encephalopathy
    cavernous sinus thrombosis

    myasthenia gravis
    thyrotoxic ophthalmolegia

Congenital squint
    latent strabismus may be exacerbated by illness in late life

Dysphagia

Neurological
    cerebrovascular accident
    motor neurone disease
    cerebral tumour – primary or secondary
    syringobulbia
    diffuse spasm
    achalasia
    disseminated sclerosis
    tetanus
    progressive supranuclear palsy

Intrinsic pharyngeal causes
    pharyngeal pouch
    foreign body

Intrinsic oesophageal causes
    carcinoma
    stricture
    oesophageal moniliasis
    Plummer–Vinson syndrome (associated with iron deficiency)
    scleroderma
    oesophageal diverticulum – **common in elderly but only rarely**
        causes dysphagia
    peptic oesophagitis

Extrinsic mechanical causes
    thyroidmegaly
    mediastinal lymphadenopathy
    bronchial carcinoma involving oesophagus
    aortic aneurysm
    left atrium dilatation

Hysteria
    a rare cause of dysphagia in the elderly

Dyspnoea

Pulmonary
    alveolar
        pneumonia
        pneumoconiosis
        bronchitis
        emphysema
    bronchial
        bronchitis
        asthma
        carcinoma
    interstitial
        extrinsic allergic alveolitis
        fibrosing alveolitis
        radiation
        uraemia
        interstitial pneumonitis
    vascular
        pulmonary embolism
        primary pulmonary hypertension
    pleural
        effusion
        pneumothorax
        mesothelioma
    mechanical
        kyphoscoliosis
        obesity
        peripheral neuropathy involving muscles of respiration
        severe ascites

Cardiac
    left ventricular failure
    pericarditis ± effusion

Miscellaneous
    anaemia
    acidosis
    hyperventilation

Anxiety state

Faecal Incontinence

constipation
diverticular disease
ischaemic colitis
ulcerative colitis
rectal prolapse
rectal carcinoma
cerebral cortex lesions – lack of inhibition
    cerebrovascular disease
    dementia
autonomic neuropathy
cord lesions
cauda equina lesions
thyrotoxicosis
carcinoid tumour
antibiotics
toxic confusional state
purgatives

Falls

History of falls given by 44% of elderly women and 24% of elderly men
Linear increase from 65–69 age group to over 85 y.

Causes
Cardiac
    arrhythmias (see p. 61)
    myocardial infarction

Pulmonary
    pulmonary embolism

Central nervous system
    transient ischaemic attack
    cerebrovascular accident
    epilepsy
    motor neurone disease
    Parkinson's and other extrapyramidal disorders
    cerebellar disorders
    labyrinthine disorders
    visual impairment
    peripheral neuropathy

Postural hypotension
    see p. 160

Gastrointestinal
    acute blood loss
    defaecation syncope

Genito-urinary
    micturition syncope

Metabolic
    myxoedema
    hypoglycaemia
    anaemia

Musculoskeletal
    muscle weakness see p. 31
    arthritis see p. 51

Drugs
    levadopa
    antidepressants
    sedatives
    phenothiazines
    alcohol
    digoxin
    antihypertensives
    diuretics

Drop attacks
    accounts for about 16–25% of falls

Miscellaneous
    tripping – single most important cause

Fatigue

anaemia
chronic infection e.g. tuberculosis, SBE
neoplasia
hypothyroidism
hyperthyroidism
Addison's disease – a rare cause
hypokalaemia
hyponatraemia
hypercalcaemia
hypocalcaemia
osteomalacia
myasthenia gravis
connective tissue disease
depression and/or anxiety
drug intoxication e.g. barbiturates, hypnotics
persistent chronic pain from any aetiology
chronic heart failure
chronic pulmonary disease
chronic renal failure

Frequency of Micturition

Renal
   urinary tract infection
   chronic renal failure
   nephritis
   renal tuberculosis

Bladder
   calculus
   detrusor instability
   prostatic enlargement
   papilloma

Miscellaneous
   hypercalcaemia
   diabetes mellitus
   diabetes insipidus
   diuretics

'Giddiness'

Special senses
    eyes – visual disturbance from any cause
    ears
        wax
        otitis media
        herpes zoster of geniculate ganglion
        labyrinthitis
        Ménière's disease

Brain stem lesions – vertebrobasilar insufficiency
Cerebellar lesions
Epilepsy
TIAs

Cardiac
    ischaemia
    arrhythmias etc.

Metabolic
    anaemia
    hypothyroidism
    hypoglycaemia etc.

Drugs
    salicylates
    quinine
    streptomycin
    psychotropic drugs

Psychogenic
Cf. postural hypotension – p. 160

Haematuria

Lower renal tract
  cystitis
  bladder papilloma
  bladder carcinoma
  bladder calculus
  bladder catheterization
      trauma
      rapid decompression
  benign prostatic hypertrophy
  prostatic carcinoma
  prostatitis
  urethritis
  urethral carcinoma

Upper renal tract
  renal calculus
  hypernephroma
  pyelonephritis
  renal vein thrombosis
  nephrosclerosis
  bacterial endocarditis
  renal infarction

Drugs
  anticoagulants

Miscellaneous
  coagulation defects secondary to
      thrombocytopaenia
      consumptive coagulopathy

pneumonia
> staphylococcal pneumonia
> Friedlander's bacillus pneumonia
> atypical pneumonia caused by *Mycoplasma pneumoniae*
> (rare)

bronchitis
bronchial carcinoma
bronchial adenoma
bronchiectasis
pulmonary tuberculosis
pulmonary infarction
pulmonary vasculitis
left ventricular failure
mitral stenosis
bleeding diathesis – secondary to
> anticoagulant therapy
> thrombocytopaenic purpura
> leukaemia

hereditary haemorrhagic telangiectasia
epistaxis presenting as haemoptysis

Hand Weakness (with wasting of muscles)

Cord lesions
    tumour
    cyst
    abscess
    motor neurone disease (see p. 128)
    trauma
    vascular lesion

Root lesions
    cervical spondylosis
    leptomeningitis of syphilis

Brachial plexus lesions
    cervical rib
    scalenus anterior
    Pancoast's tumour

Nerve lesions
    median nerve – **carpal tunnel syndrome**
    ulnar nerve lesions
    polyneuropathy

Muscular
    dystrophia myotonia
    ischaemic myositis
    'shoulder-hand syndrome'

Miscellaneous
    arthritis affecting hand e.g. rheumatoid arthritis
    'parietal wasting'

Headache

Temporal arteritis
meningitis
subarachnoid haemorrhage
intracerebral haemorrhage
cerebral thrombosis
cerebral abscess
cerebral tumour – primary or secondary
trigeminal neuralgia
cervical spondylosis

Eyes
glaucoma
iritis

sinusitis

Skull
Paget's disease
tumour involving the skull
osteomyelitis of skull
dental pain

depression
(any severe medical illness may produce headache although this
is a less common presentation in the elderly)

Jaundice

Liver
   viral hepatitis see p. 188
   septicaemia
   carcinoma – primary or **secondary**
   cirrhosis – 'senile cirrhosis', primary biliary cirrhosis, cryptogenic
      cirrhosis, cirrhosis secondary to haemochromatosis etc.

Biliary tree
   stone
   carcinoma – **head of pancreas,** ampullary or bile duct
   porta hepatis lymph node enlargement (usually from car-
      cinoma)
   biliary stricture
   infective cholangitis
   sclerosing cholangitis
   duodenal diverticulum

Cardiac/Pulmonary
   congestive heart failure
   pulmonary infarction
   pneumonia occasionally

Drugs
   see p. 100

Miscellaneous
   haemolysis
   ulcerative colitis
   hereditary unconjugated hyperbilirubinaemia

Leg Ulcers

varicose veins
peripheral vascular disease ± trauma
pressure sores
burns
neuropathy ± trauma
ulcerating gouty tophi
pemphigus
pemphigoid

Tumours
    basal cell carcinoma
    melanoma
    mycosis fungoides
    squamous cell carcinoma

Vasculitis
    rheumatoid arthritis
    polyarteritis nodosa
    giant cell arteritis

    dysproteinaemias

Drugs – steroids
    pyoderma gangrenosum – associated with ulcerative colitis or
      Crohn's disease
    frost bite

Leg Weakness

Muscle
: polymyositis

Neuromuscular
: **Eaton-Lambert syndrome (myasthenic syndrome)**
myasthenia gravis (occasionally)

Nerve
: polyneuropathy – see p. 153
Guillain–Barré syndrome
cord lesion
cauda equina lesion
motor neurone disease
DS
cerebrovascular accident
cerebral tumour
common peroneal nerve palsy

Metabolic
: **osteomalacia**
Cushing's disease
hypokalaemia

Drugs
: steroids
neomycin
phenothiazines
carbenoxolone
diphenylhydantoins

Miscellaneous
: **arthritis**
Parkinson's disease
depression
any severe generalized illness
prolonged immobility

Low Back Pain

Degeneration of spine (disc, ligaments etc.)
osteoporosis
osteomalacia
Paget's disease
tumours arising from the spine
secondary involvement by tumours of the spine
lymphoma involving the spine
osteomylitis
renal pain
pancreatitis
pancreatic carcinoma
pressure sores
herpes zoster
psychogenic
pelvic disorders

Muscle Weakness

Muscle disease
    polymyositis see p. 71
    myasthenia gravis
        autoimmune
        muscles fatigue on exertion
        ocular and bulbar muscles usually involved
        Tensilon test positive
        treatment – anticholinesterases, steroids or ACTH
    Eaton–Lambert syndrome
        myasthenic myopathic disorder
        associated with carcinoma (oat cell usually)
        proximal muscles commonly involved
        facial muscles less commonly involved
        muscle power improves transiently with exercise
        tendon reflexes depressed
        Tensilon test may be positive but usually it is negative
        no response to anticholinesterases; respond to guanidine
            hydrochloride
    Trichinosis
    ischaemia
    dystrophia myotonia

Neurological
    neuropathy see p. 153
    cerebrovascular disease
    motor neurone disease
    polio

Metabolic/Endocrine
    osteomalacia
    Cushing's disease
    hypokalaemia
    thyrotoxicosis
    ectopic production of ACTH
    hypocalcaemia
    hypothyroidism with pseudomyotonia

Joints
    secondary to generalized severe arthritis – see p. 51

Drugs
    carbenoxolone
    steroids
    diuretics

Drugs (*continued*)
>   diphenylhydantoin
>   neomycin
>   procainamide
>   phenothiazines
>   tetracyclines
>   sulphonamide

Miscellaneous
>   **any cause of immobility** – see p. 116
>   prolonged catabolic state

Nausea and Vomiting

Oesophagus
    hiatus hernia with oesophagitis

Stomach
    peptic ulcer
    gastritis
    carcinoma
    volvulus

Intestine
    enteritis
    obstruction from any cause
    sigmoid volvulus
    constipation

Metabolic
    diabetic coma
    hypercalcaemia
    renal failure
    liver failure

Miscellaneous
    cholecystitis
    pancreatitis
    hepatitis
    pyelonephritis
    pneumonia
    meningitis
    labyrinthitis
    cerebral tumour – primary or secondary
    myocardial infarction
    congestive cardiac failure

Drugs
    digoxin
    diamorphine
    levadopa
    spironolactone
    antibiotics

Non-specific Illness

malignant disease
tuberculosis
bacterial endocarditis
depression
renal failure
anaemia
hypothyroidism
temporal arteritis
osteomalacia
bereavement
drug intoxication e.g. barbiturates
collagen vascular disease
apathetic thyrotoxicosis
Addison's disease

Oedema (peripheral)

Cardiac
    congestive cardiac failure secondary to
        ischaemia
        pericarditis
        valvular lesions
        pulmonary emboli
        chronic lung disease
        cardiomyopathies

Vascular
    venous thrombosis – idiopathic or secondary to polycythaemia,
        dysproteinaemias, tumour etc.
    incompetent valves – varicose veins
    cellulitis involving legs
    immobility

Lymphatic obstruction
    neoplastic
    congenital
    post-cellulitis

Hepatic failure from any cause

Renal
    nephrotic syndrome

Miscellaneous
    low serum albumin
        poor diet
        excessive loss from gut

Drugs
    steroids
    carbenoxolone
    indomethacin
    phenylbutazone
    oestrogens, etc.

Painful Red Eye

Lid
    abscess
    stye

Conjunctiva
    foreign body
    conjunctivitis

Cornea
    ulcer
        traumatic
        herpetic
    keratitis
    foreign body

Iris/aqueous
    acute glaucoma
    uveitis

Pruritus

Skin conditions
    eczema
    pemphigoid
    pediculosis
    erythroderma associated with psoriasis, **mycosis fungoides** etc.
    senile pruritis

Drugs
    with allergic rash
        penicillin
        cotrimoxazole, etc.
    with no rash
        morphine
        chlorpromazine etc.
        testosterone

Haematological causes
    Hodgkin's disease
    lymphomas
    iron deficiency anaemia
    polycythaemia

Metabolic
    diabetes mellitus
    hyperthyroidism
    hypothyroidism

Obstructive jaundice
    stone
    tumour at head of pancreas
    cholestatic jaundice
        primary biliary cirrhosis
        drugs see p. 100

Chronic renal failure

Malignancy
    particularly abdominal carcinomas

Speech Disturbance

Dysarthria
    brain stem lesions
    cerebellar lesions
    motor neurone disease
    myasthenia gravis
    Parkinson's disease
    oro-facial dyskinesia
    alcohol
    badly fitting dentures
    Steele–Richardson syndrome

Dysphasia
    cerebrovascular accident
    malignancy – primary or secondary
    temporal lobe abscess
    neurosyphylis
    Alzheimer's disease

Hoarseness
    laryngitis
    laryngeal polyp or carcinoma
    myxoedema
    rheumatoid arthritis affecting the cricoarytenoid joint
    systemic diseases affecting the larynx
        amyloid
        diabetes mellitus
        collagen disease
    psychogenic

Swelling of Glands (Lymphadenopathy)

Malignancy
>lymphomas
>leukaemias
>secondaries from other malignancies

Infection
>any infection may cause swelling
>specific
>>tuberculosis
>>toxoplasmosis
>>infectious mononucleosis

granulomatous conditions
rheumatoid arthritis
SLE
amyloid

Drugs
>barbiturates
>salicylates
>nalidixic acid
>phenytoin
>PAS

Ear
  wax
  otitis media
  otosclerosis
  acoustic neuroma
  Ménière's syndrome
  labyrinthitis
  drugs
      streptomycin
      quinine
      salicylates

Cerebral
  cerebral tumour
  epilepsy

Brainstem
  vertebrobasilar insufficiency

psychogenic
  tinnitus may be part of hallucinations

pulsating tinnitus
  A/V malformation

Tremor

Resting or static
    Parkinson's disease – 'pill rolling'

Action
    anxiety – coarse tremor
    thyrotoxicosis – fine tremor of outstretched hands
    drug intoxication
        alcohol
        barbiturate withdrawal, etc.
    benign or essential – can be familial
    senile – fine and rapid – at late stages can be present at rest
    intention tremor – tremor increases at end of movement – present in cerebellar disease, MS, etc.
    flapping or 'wing beating' – characteristic of liver failure but it can be present in respiratory or renal failure
    hysteria – can be fine or coarse

Visual Failure

Lens
 cataract
Cornea
 keratitis
 keratomalacia
Iris
 uveitis
Aqueous
 glaucoma
Vitreous
 haemorrhage
Optic nerve
 compression
 demyelinating disease
Retina
 detachment
 optic neuritis
 retinal artery thrombosis
 retinal vein thrombosis
 papilloedema
 optic nerve atrophy
 macular degeneration
 temporal arteritis
 choroid retinitis
Intracerebral
 pituitary tumours
 damage to chiasma at pituitary surgery
 intracranial tumours
 cerebrovascular accident
 intracerebral abscess
 raised intracranial pressure from any cause
 aneurysm
Cranial
 trauma
 Paget's disease

Orbital lesions

Drugs
 chloroquine
 practolol

Common disorders

Anaemia

WHO definition: Hb $<13\,g/dl$ in men and $<12\,g/dl$ in women
Occurs in 5-20% of elderly
Iron deficiency anaemia
    aetiology
        poor nutrition
        poverty, immobility etc. (inability to get food)
        defective absorbtion
            gastritis
            partial or total gastrectomy
            steatorrhoea see p. 207
        excessive loss of iron (blood loss)
            oesophagitis
            peptic ulceration
            gastric carcinoma
            colonic diverticuli
            colonic or caecal carcinoma
            rectal
                haemorrhoids
                polyp
                carcinoma
            vaginal bleeding (carcinoma of cervix
              or uterus)
            haematuria
                bladder papilloma
                carcinoma
                hypernephroma etc.
      Drugs
            salicylates
            steroids
            indomethacin
            phenylbutazone

    investigations
        serum iron↓
        TIBC↑
        MCV↓
        MCHC↓

    clinical features
        pallor
        glossitis
        low grade fever

confusion
falls
congestive heart failure
Plummer–Vinson syndrome
koilonychia

treatment
oral iron
ferrous sulphate 200 mg t.d.s.
ferrous gluconate 300 mg t.d.s.
**if patient unable or unwilling to take oral iron: total dose
i.v. infusion used** (dose: 4.5 mg iron-dextran/kg body
weight/g Hb deficient)
test dose given before the infusion to avoid serious allergic
reaction

Megaloblastic Anaemias

B_{12} deficiency anaemia
aetiology
poor diet
pernicious anaemia – incidence 1% after age of 60
partial or total gastrectomy
atrophic gastritis
carcinoma of stomach
jejunal diverticular disease (stagnant loop syndrome)
ileal resection
malabsorption see p. 127
metformin

clinical features
signs of anaemia
yellow tinge to skin
pyrexia
glossitis
anorexia
in severe cases
hepatosplenomegaly
heart failure
haemorrhages in retina

complications
    peripheral neuropathy
    dementia
    subacute combined degeneration

investigations
    MCV↑
    macrocytosis
    megaloblasts in bone marrow
    hypersegmented polymorphs
    in pernicious anaemia
        Schilling's test + ve
        parietal cell antibodies
        intrinsic factor antibodies

treatment
    B_{12} 500 μg initially followed by 250 μg of cyanocobalamin
        at monthly intervals

Folate deficiency anaemia
    aetiology

poor diet　⎤　**account for majority of folate**
malabsorption　⎦　**deficiency in elderly**

increased demand
    lymphoma
    neoplasm
    infection
liver disease
drugs
    phenytoin etc.

clinical features
    changes of megaloblastic anaemia
    red cell folate <100 μg/ml packed cells
    may be associated with
        mild confusion
        irritability
        depression
        dementia
        peripheral neuropathy
        features resembling subacute combined degeneration of B_{12} deficiency

treatment
    folic acid 5 mg/day

Sideroblastic anaemia
    hypochromic anaemia with ring sideroblasts in bone marrow
        (sideroblasts – erythroblasts with >5 iron granules)
    impaired iron utilization
    acquired form can be
        primary
            serum iron normal
            TIBC often reduced
        secondary to
            myeloproliferative disorder
            myeloma
            carcinoma
            collagen disease
            myxoedema
            drugs
                antituberculous
                phenacetin
                chloramphenicol

treatment
    pyridoxine ± folic acid
    treatment of primary condition producing it
    blood transfusion for symptomatic relief – in refractory
        cases repeated blood transfusions may be necessary

Anaemia of chronic disease
    normochromic normocytic anaemia
    haematinics of little value

aetiology
    tuberculosis
    diverticulitis
    rheumatoid arthritis
    pressure sores
    malignancy (anaemia associated with malignancy can also
        be iron deficiency anaemia or leukoerythroblastic
        anaemia)
    hypothyroidism (may also be associated with iron deficien-
        cy or B_{12} deficiency)
    renal failure

Hypoplastic anaemia
    uncommon in elderly
    ↓red cell production ±↓ white cells and platelets

    aetiology
        idiopathic
            senile hypoplastic anaemia
            myeloma
            myeloproliferative disorders
            neoplasia
            paroxysmal nocturnal haemoglobulinuria associated
                with thymoma
            drugs
                cytotoxic agents
                antibiotics e.g. chloramphenicol, sulphona-
                    mides, penicillin etc.
                phenylbutazone
                phenytoin
                tolbutamide, chlorpropamide
                quinidine
                chlorthiazide
                carbamazepine
                oestrogens

    clinical features
        insidious onset
        symptoms and signs of anaemia
        bleeding if platelets reduced
        repeated infections common

    diagnosis
        pancytopenia, reticulocyte count low
        bone marrow
            hypoplastic in idiopathic and in those with anaemia
                secondary to drugs
            in others marrow also shows changes of the primary
                condition

    treatment
        supportive therapy e.g. blood transfusions
        anabolic steroids
        androgens (fluoxymesterone 20–40 mg/day) may help

Haemolytic anaemia
    aetiology
        idiopathic autoimmune haemolytic anaemia
        reticulosis
        leukaemias
        paroxysmal nocturnal haemoglobulinuria
        drugs
            methyldopa, quinine etc.

    clinical features
        anaemia
        reticulocyte count ↑
        unconjugated hyperbilirubinaemia
        urobilinogen in urine
        warm antibodies in case of idiopathic AHA – Coomb's +ve

    treatment
        blood transfusion
        steroids – prednisone 60 mg/day reducing quickly to
            maintenance dose
        azathioprine – used if dosage of steroid required to control
            disease is very high

Arthritis

Osteoarthritis
> **commonest arthritis**
> **80% over 60 years of age have some changes of OA**
> degenerative joint disease characterized by loss of joint cartilage and osteophytes
> can be primary or secondary (trauma, infection, rheumatoid arthritis, avascular necrosis etc.)
> asymmetrical seronegative arthritis
> clinical features vary according to joint(s) involved and severity of the disease but pain and restriction of movement common

> hands
>> terminal I/P joints commonly involved (Heberdon's node)
>> Bouchard's node – proximal IP joint lesion
>> M/P joints commonly involved in rheumatoid arthritis are not usually affected by osteoarthritis

> spine
>> cervical spondylosis – see p. 65
>> lumbar spine
>>> local back pain
>>> nerve root pain due to pressure of osteophytes

> **hip**
>> **may present with pain in groin or in knees (referred)**
>> **pain and restriction of movements may lead to immobility and falls**

> knees
>> early symptoms are pain and stiffness
>> later genu varum deformity may develop
>> effusion ± loose bodies may be present
>> effusion may lead to synovial cyst (Baker's cyst)

> occasionally elderly may present with acute and transient inflammatory joint disease particularly involving the hands

> treatment
>> reassurance
>> analgesics for pain
>> local heat for mild cases

physiotherapy – important
>   for improving movement of joints
>   for improving and maintaining muscular strength
>   may require regular or intermittent therapy on day
>   hospital basis to keep patient mobile and at home

surgery for
>   debridement
>   removal of loose bodies
>   osteotomy or total joint replacement e.g. for knees

Crystalline arthritis
>   gout
>>   idiopathic or associated with myeloma, lymphoma etc.
>>   monoarticular arthritis
>>   high incidence in females
>>   raised uric acid may be found
>>   uric acid crystals (negatively birefringent) may be detected
>>   in synovial fluid
>>   acute attack may be precipitated by thiazide diuretics
>>   rapid response to colchicine (0.5–1 mg 2-hourly until relief
>>   is achieved), phenylbutazone or indomethacin
>>   recurrent attacks may be prevented by probenecid or
>>   allopurinol (used especially if renal failure also present)

pseudogout
>   chondrocalcinosis
>   +ve birefringent calcium pyrophosphate crystals found on
>   microscopy of synovial fluid
>   may be associated with hyperparathyroidism and
>   haemochromatosis
>   X-rays – articular calcification may be seen especially in
>   the knees
>   predilection for larger joints
>   treatment
>>   of acute attack – phenylbutazone 600 mg daily,
>>   reduce the dose as symptoms improve
>>   in between attacks – analgesics (as for OA)

Rheumatoid arthritis – see p. 74

Psoriasis
Ankylosing spondylitis
Ulcerative colitis
Polyarteritis nadosa
SLE
Stevens–Johnson syndrome

Miscellaneous
    hypertrophic pulmonary osteoarthropathy
        associated with malignancy (bronchogenic)
        finger clubbing
        arthralgia
        X-rays – increased thickness of periosteum of distal
           forearm bones
        treatment – analgesics, tumour resection or vagotomy

    polyarthritis associated with carcinoma of breast, prostate,
        bladder etc.
    infective arthritis
        pyogenic (staphylococcus, streptococcus, pneumococcus,
           tuberculosis etc.)
        predisposing factors
           damaged joint
           local steroid injection
        diagnosis made on culture of blood and synovial fluid
        treatment
           according to organism and its sensitivity (but treat-
             ment with penicillin and cloxacillin is started at
             time of diagnosis and treatment is altered when
             the bacteriological results come back)
           repeated aspirations
           immobilization for 1–2 weeks
           intensive physiotherapy after that

Asthma

Definition: A state characterized by partial airways obstruction, reversible spontaneously or as a result of treatment

Types
    intrinsic – late onset – common type seen in the elderly
    extrinsic – allergic

Prevalence – 6.5%

Clinical features
    dyspnoea
    paroxysmal cough
    chest tightness
    wheezing
    symptoms made worse by emotional factors
    $FEV_1/FVC\downarrow$
    may have eosinophilia in sputum or blood
    may have positive family history

Treatment
    bronchodilators
        salbutamol 2–4 mg q.d.s. ± salbutamol inhaler two puffs
            four times a day
        aminophylline suppositories at night for night time
            bronchospasm
        parenteral salbutamol in acute attack
    steroids
        indicated
        if symptoms do not settle with bronchodilators
        in acute attack
    if steroids are necessary to keep patient symptom-free try
        ACTH or inhaled beclomethasone (200 mg q.d.s.) – both
        have low risk with regard to adrenal suppression

    NB side effects of steroids
        iatrogenic Cushing's disease
        confusion, psychoses
        osteoporosis
        liability to severe infections
        diabetes mellitus
        gastric ulcer
        cataract

raised intracranial pressure
skin fragility
fluid retention

Intal
useful in extrinsic asthma; also in some intrinsic cases

NB as in the case of beclomethasone inhaler elderly may find it difficult to use the Intal inhaler: they have to be shown many times how to use these inhalers
antibiotic
for associated infection in acute attack

Atypical Pneumonias

Mycoplasma pneumoniae
    aetiology
        Mycoplasma pneumoniae = Eaton's agent
    clinical features
        fever
        malaise
        cough
        sore throat
        confusion
        haemoptysis in some cases
        fine rales on chest examination – but not impressive
        ESR high in $^2/_3$
        X-rays
            extensive bilateral lower lobe involvement
            less dense (fluffy) changes than seen in bacterial
                infection
            radiological changes are more than one would expect
                from clinical examination
        cold agglutinins +ve in about 90%

    treatment
        tetracycline 250 mg q.d.s.
        erythromycin 1.5 g/day

Legionnaire's disease
    named after an outbreak at convention of American Legion-
    naires in Philadelphia in 1976

    aetiology
        legionnaire's bacillus (*Legionella pneumophila*)

    clinical features
        illness begins with
            malaise
            myalgia
            headache
            fever $>39°C$
            pain in chest
            pain in abdomen
            confusion
        in some progresses in few days to
            shock

                respiratory failure
                renal failure
                GIT bleeding
            others recover spontaneously
            mortality 17–25%

investigations
        WCC 5–15 × 10^9/litre
        serum sodium tends to be low
        liver function tests – abnormal
        chest X-rays
                patchy interstitial infiltrations or consolidated areas
                occasionally effusions
diagnosis made by
        serology – indirect fluorescent antibody test
        culturing bacillus from sputum

treatment
        erythromycin or tetracycline

Bronchiectasis

Definition: widening and distortion of bronchi

Incidence: 13% at autopsy, 3.5% in clinical studies

Aetiology – may develop
    following suppurative pneumonia
    following pneumonia complicating measles or whooping cough
    following obstruction of bronchus by carcinoma

Clinical features
    chronic productive cough
    sputum +++
    recurrent chest infections
    haemoptysis
    classical signs of finger clubbing, cyanosis, coarse crepitations
      are only rarely found
    diagnosis made on bronchography although plain chest X-rays
      may suggest its presence

Complications
    severe haemoptysis leading to anaemia
    cerebral abscess
    empyema

Treatment
    antibiotics for acute exacerbations of infections
    physiotherapy – postural drainage – very important
    transfusion if severe anaemia present
    on rare occasions surgery may help if bronchiectasis is localized
      and causing chronic ill-health.

Bullous Diseases

Pemphigus vulgaris
    thin walled blisters
    intra-epidermal
    axillae and groin involved commonly
    increased incidence in Jews
    Nikolsky's sign +ve
    secondary infection common
    anaemia
    electrolyte imbalance
    treatment
        steroids – prednisone 60–80 mg/day – reducing quickly to
            maintenance dose of 10–20 mg/day
        azathioprine if steroids not effective
        antibiotic e.g. tetracycline for secondary infection

Pemphigoid
    80% of cases are over 60 years of age
    itchy thick walled blisters
    may contain blood
    symmetrical over limbs and abdomen
    anti-basement membrane antibodies
    Nikolsky's sign –ve
    may have underlying malignancy
    treatment
        steroids – smaller dosage than in case of pemphigus is
            required

Benign familial chronic pemphigus = Hailey–Hailey disease
    autosomal dominant
    vesicles in axilla, groin etc.
    skin biopsy: extensive acantholysis, suprabasal split
    heat worsens condition
    cold produces remission
    prognosis good

Stevens–Johnson syndrome
    aetiology
        infection
            herpes simplex
            mycoplasma
        drugs
            sulphonamides
            barbiturates etc.

bullous eruption
fever
malaise
confusion
mucosal involvement (mouth, genitalia, rectum)
treatment
    prednisone 30–40 mg/day for those with constitutional
      upset
    antibiotics if secondary infection develops

Cardiac Arrhythmias

Atrial fibrillation
- commonest arrhythmia in the elderly after ectopics
- 10–15% patients admitted to hospital have this arrhythmia
- atrial rate 360+ per minute
- irregularly irregular pulse

aetiology
- **ischaemic heart disease**
- **thyrotoxicosis**
- hypertension
- myocarditis
- cardiomyopathy
- **respiratory infections**
- pericarditis
- mitral valve disease
- atrial involvement in malignant disease
- **idiopathic**

treatment
- digoxin – **loading dose 0.5-0.75/mg followed by maintenance dose of 0.0625-0.25/mg per day – maintenance dose depends largely on renal function**
- DC cardioversion occasionally used if aetiological factor removed
- **NB digitalis toxicity may present with**
    - **nausea, vomiting, anorexia**
    - **confusion**
    - xanthopsia
    - gynaecomastia
    - **arrhythmias, including heart block**
    - **in case of suspected toxicity, measure serum digoxin level at least 6 hours post-dose**

Atrial flutter
- atrial rate 260–320 per minute
- pulse regular unless varying degree of block
- flutter waves in JVP and ECG

aetiology – as for atrial fibrillation

treatment – as for atrial fibrillation

Supraventricular tachycardia
        pulse regular unless varying degrees of block
        atrial rate 160–200 per minute
        may slow on
                carotid sinus pressure **(NB atheromatous vessels)**
                valsalva manoeuvre
                orbit pressure **(NB retinal detachment)**

        treatment
                β-blocking drugs
                digoxin
                verapamil
                DC cardioversion

Heart block
        first degree – prolongation of PR interval (>0.2 ms) – 2% of
                elderly show some prolongation of PR interval
        second degree –
                Mobitz type I (Wenkebach phenomenon)
                Mobitz type II
        third degree – complete AV dissociation
        NB can occur in presence of atrial fibrillation or atrial flutter

        aetiology
                myocardial infarction
                myocardial ischaemia
                idiopathic fibrosis of conducting tissue
                infective endocarditis
                hypertension
                sarcoidosis
                myocarditis
                cardiomyopathy
                drugs: especially digoxin

        clinical features
                asymptomatic to syncope (Stokes–Adams attack)
                bradycardia usually present in 3rd degree block
                rate depends on level of block

        treatment
                if asymptomatic – none

to increase ventricular rate temporarily –
atropine 0.6 mg parenterally, may be repeated
isoprenaline 2–4 mg in 500 ml slowly i.v.
corticosteroids – may be of temporary value post–MI
sustained-release isoprenaline, 30–120 mg 8 hourly,
increasing to maximum of 360 mg per day
pacemaker – obligatory if syncope occurs or if medical
therapy fails

Sick sinus syndrome or bradycardia-tachycardia syndrome

Sinus node dysfunction

clinical features
sinus bradycardia
sinus arrest
junctional escape beats
tachycardias
varying degrees of block
dizziness
fall
chest pain
dyspnoea
stroke (secondary to emboli or hypotension)

aetiology
diffuse coronary artery disease

treatment
drugs usually of little benefit and may be hazardous
pacemaker essential

Ventricular tachycardia

120–200 per minute
P waves unrelated to ventricular complexes
QRS complexes broad and often bizarre
slightly irregular rhythm
hypotension
shock

treatment
>cardiac monitoring of all therapy
>DC cardioversion
>lignocaine i.v. 100 mg initially
>disopyramide i.v. 2 mg/kg bolus then 200 mg b.d. or t.d.s.
>β-blockers
>>propranolol i.v. 1 mg over 1 minute – up to 10 mg
>>practolol – 10 mg i.v. slowly

Ventricular fibrillation

>follow: ventricular tachycardia
>R on T ectopic beat
>cf. Stokes–Adams attack
>circulatory arrest
>pulse not palpable
>ECG – irregular complexes of varying shapes and sizes

>treatment
>>direct current shock + lignocaine

Cervical Spondylosis

Degenerative disease of cervical spine

Prevalence: 72% over age 70
Clinical features
    stiff neck
    root compression symptoms and signs
        pain
        weakness and atrophy of hand muscles
        absent or reduced reflexes in the upper limb
    vertebro-basilar insufficiency
    cervical myelopathy
        commonest cause of cord compression in the elderly
        weakness and wasting in upper limb and UMN signs in
          lower limbs with extensor plantars
        CSF protein may be raised
        Queckenstedt's test +ve at lumbar puncture
        myelogram may be necessary in these patients to exclude
          other compressive lesions
    X-rays
        narrowing of intervertebral spaces (C_6–C_7 most frequently
          shows this)
        osteophytes
        reduced diameter of neural canal in some

Treatment
    cervical collar and analgesia for root compression
    diazepam if tension present in muscles
    physiotherapy once pain has subsided
    surgery – decompression in selected cases may prevent progres-
        sion of leg weakness

Chronic Brain Syndrome (Dementia)

Incidence: 5-10% in general population over 65

Aetiology
> **degeneration**
>> associated with neurone loss, plaques, neurofibrillary tangles and granular vacuolar degeneration
>> Pick's disease, Alzheimer's disease
>> Huntingdon's chorea
>> Jacob–Creutzfeldt
> **cerebrovascular disease**
>> atherosclerosis
>> giant cell arteritis
> infection – encephalitis, syphilis, meningitis, intracerebral abscess
> **malignancy**
>> cerebral tumours e.g. meningioma
>> non-metastatic complication
> **metabolic**
>> anoxia
>> B_{12} deficiency
>> hypothyroidism
>> liver failure
>> pellagra
>> prolonged hypoglycaemia
>> hypercalcaemia
> **drugs**
>> **long-term barbiturate ingestion**
>> alcohol (Wernicke's encephalopathy)
> **subdural haematoma** – see p. 177
> **normal pressure hydrocephalus** – see p. 141
> miscellaneous
>> multiple sclerosis
>> post-traumatic
> **cf. 'pseudodementia' of depression** – see p. 84

Clinical features
> earliest sign may be loss of interest
> inability to perform daily activities of living
> memory poor for recent events
> concentration poor
> exaggerated emotions – lability common

social and character deterioration
    self-neglect
    antisocial behaviour
    incontinence etc.
paranoid delusions and hallucinations may occur
steplike deterioration and focal signs in arteriosclerotic
    dementia

Specific investigations
    serum B_{12}
    T_4
    serology
    skull X-rays + computer-assisted tomography if subdural,
        tumour or normal pressure hydrocephalus suspected

Management
    difficult
    maintain at home those who are not very confused with sup-
        ports like day hospital, district nurse, home help etc.
    for those unable to look after themselves at home –
        LARC if not too agitated or confused
        psychiatric hospital or unit for elderly mentally infirm if
            patient very confused
        geriatric hospital for those with associated severe physical
            disease
    drug therapy – for anxiety and agitation
        thioridazine 10 mg t.d.s.
        promazine 25 mg t.d.s.
        chlorpromazine 50–150 mg t.d.s. or q.d.s.
        diazepam 2–10 mg t.d.s.
        doses of each adjusted according to response
        for sleep use dichloralphenazone
        thyroxine for myxoedema
        B_{12} for those with deficiency of B_{12}
        antidepressants if depression present

Chronic Obstructive Airways Disease

Emphysema
>definition: dilatation of air spaces distal to terminal bronchioles with destruction of their walls

>two types
>>panacinar
>>centrilobular

>clinical features
>>more common in males
>>underweight
>>breathlessness
>>scanty sputum
>>'pink puffer'
>>lip pursing
>>use of accessory muscles of respiration
>>chest X-rays – flat diaphragm; vertical heart; large retrosternal translucent space; bullae in $^1/_3$

>complications
>>pneumothorax
>>respiratory failure

>treatment
>>stop smoking
>>no specific treatment
>>control of infection
>>for respiratory failure see p. 169

Chronic bronchitis

>definition
>>mucoid sputum and cough for at least three months of a year for two or more years
>>smoking probably the most important aetiological factor

>clinical features
>>acute exacerbations with varying degrees of airway obstruction
>>'blue bloater'
>>cor pulmonale common

treatment
    for acute exacerbation
        controlled oxygen
        physiotherapy
        antibiotics
        bronchodilators
    for respiratory failure see p. 169

NB intermediate type of chronic obstructive airways disease most common

Colitis

Ischaemic colitis
 aetiology
  atherosclerosis
  arteritis
  embolism – atrial fibrillation, myocardial infarction, SBE
   etc.

 clinical features
  abdominal pain
  diarrhoea
  blood in stools
  vomiting, pyrexia and confusion may accompany acute
   onset
  acute occlusion
   peritonitis
   perforation
  X-rays – barium enema may show thumb printing, saw
   tooth appearance and/or sacculation due to formation
   of pseudodiverticulae

 treatment
  treat the underlying cause
  subacute attack without occlusion requires no treatment
   as it tends to settle spontaneously in 2–4 weeks
  surgery for stricture or massive mesenteric occlusion or
   perforation

Ulcerative colitis
 aetiology
  multifactorial – genetic, autoimmune, infection etc.

 clinical features
  diarrhoea or constipation
  blood or slime in motion
  weight loss
  anaemia
  fever
  confusion
  general ill-health
  arthralgia, arthritis
  episcleritis, iritis
  erythema nodosum
  pyoderma gangrenosum
  hepatic and biliary dysfunction

complications
    perforation
    acute dilatation
    carcinoma
    pericholangitis

investigations
    sigmoidoscopy – uniformly granular mucosa
    rectal biopsy
    barium enema
        lack of haustration (may also be seen in Crohn's
            colitis)
        mucosal ulceration
        polypoid projections

treatment
    retention hydrocortisone enemas – especially for mild colitis
        and proctitis
    systemic steroids if enemas not successful
    sulphasalazine (0.5 g q.d.s.) to prevent relapse
    surgery indicated for
        toxic dilatation
        failure of medical treatment
        carcinoma
        prophylaxis of carcinoma

Pseudomembranous colitis
    aetiology – *Clostridia difficile*
    clinical features
        usually follow antibiotic administration
            lincomycin
            clindamycin
            chlortetracycline
            ampicillin
            cotrimoxazole etc.
        diarrhoea leading to dehydration and shock
        mortality rate in elderly high (70%)
        toxic dilatation as in ulcerative colitis may occur

    proctoscopy
        ulceration with mucosal plaques
        ulceration initially may be patchy
    isolation of *Cl. difficile* or its toxin from the stools

management
    stop antibiotics
    parenteral hydration
    vancomycin 125–500 mg q.d.s.
    steroids

**prevention: use antibiotics in elderly with caution i.e. only
when necessary**

Collagen Vascular Diseases

Dermatomyositis
- skin rash: on face, anterior chest, elbows, knees
- muscle
    - proximal muscle weakness
    - pain and tenderness less common
    - muscle biopsy – necrosis and infiltration by chronic inflammatory cells
- ½ have polyarthralgia or arthritis
- Raynaud's phenomenon
- associated with malignancy (50%)
- plasma levels of CPK and SGOT may be high
- treatment
    - steroids – prednisone 30–40 mg/day until improvement occurs
    - immunosuppressives if steroids fail

Lupus erythematosus
- **presents insidiously in the elderly**
- **large number present with localized form**
- **in elderly it is often drug-precipitated**
- skin
    - facial erythema
    - telangiectasia over nail bed
- ESR↑
- leukopenia
- LE cells (80%)
- ANF +ve
- anti-DNA antibodies +ve
- complications – any organ can be affected but kidney involvement common
- treatment
    - steroids – prednisone 100 mg/day may be required if disease severe
    - azathioprine
    - cyclophosphamide
- localized form
    - common in females
    - face, scalp, upper trunk etc. involved
    - LE cells only occasionally seen
    - treatment not required
- (cf. SLE-like syndrome-associated with hydrallazine, procainamide etc.)
    - dose related
    - renal involvement uncommon

Rheumatoid arthritis
    may present as
        quiescent arthritis
        continuing arthritis
        acute arthritis – $1/3$ **present in this manner,** onset often abrupt
    common in females
    morning stiffness
    multiple joint involvement common – monoarthritis a rare presentation
    ESR↑
    high titre of rheumatoid factor common in large numbers
    erosions and nodules less common than in younger patients
    extra-articular complications
        anaemia – very common
        vasculitis
        skin ulceration
        neuropathy – rare in the elderly
        mesenteric infarction
    important problems in the elderly
        immobility
        falls
        pressure sores
        septic arthritis
        complications of treatment
    Treatment
        rest for acute stage
        anti-inflammatory agents (e.g. aspirin, indomethacin, ibuprofen, naproxen etc.)
        steroids for acute attack – intra-articular injection used if one joint particularly involved more than others
        if no response with steroids use gold or chloroquine, or penicillamine or immunosuppression
        iron for iron deficiency anaemia
        surgery
            tendon repair
            correction of deformity especially in hands
            osteotomy
            arthroplasty used especially in case of knee and hip
            nerve entrapment syndromes

rehabilitation (physiotherapy and occupational therapy) is an important part of treatment of elderly with rheumatoid arthritis if problems like immobility, falls and pressure sores are to be prevented.

Scleroderma
- disorder of connective tissue
- common in females
- skin tight over hands and face (skin tethering)
- fingers become tapered (atrophy and resorption)
- weight loss
- Raynaud's phenomenom
- may involve
  - oesophagus (becomes atonic)
  - lung
  - heart
  - bowel
- localized form – morphea
- CRST syndrome (calcinosis, Raynaud's, sclerodactyly and telangiectasia) – a variant of scleroderma
- treatment
  - no specific treatment available
  - physiotherapy
  - protection of extremities

Colonic Diverticular Disease

Incidence: **50% over age 80 by barium enema**

Aetiology
    ? lack of fibre in diet

Clinical features
    asymptomatic
    pain in left iliac fossa (78%)
    tenderness in left iliac fossa
    constipation (35%)
    diarrhoea (19%)
    nausea
    flatulence (13%)
    rectal bleeding (30%)

Complications
    diverticulitis
    haemorrhage
    abscess formation
    perforation
        peritonitis
        pericolic abscess
        fistula into other viscera, especially bladder or vagina
    anaemia

Treatment
    usually medical
    high residue diet
    bulk laxative
    anticholinergic drugs (best avoided in elderly because of side-effects)
    surgery: sigmoid myotomy has produced good results in selected cases; resection of involved segment rarely
    antimicrobial drugs should be reserved for diverticulitis

Confusion (Toxic confusional state)

Aetiology
    infections
        pneumonia (bacterial or viral), urinary tract infection, septicaemia, meningitis, encephalitis, infected ulcers, diverticulitis, tuberculosis
    cardiac
        ischaemia
        myocardial infarction
        arrhythmias
        subacute bacterial endocarditis
    cerebrovascular disease
        stroke (CVA)
        transient ischaemic attacks (TIA's)
    trauma
        subdural
        fracture of bone, particularly femur
    tumours
        cerebral primary tumours as well as secondary tumours
        non-metastatic complication
    metabolic
        hyponatraemia
        hypokalaemia
        hypocalcaemia
        hypoglycaemia
        ketoacidosis
        hypercalcaemia
        liver, renal or respiratory failure
        thyrotoxicosis
          hypothyroidism
        chronic anaemia
    drugs
        amitriptyline
        anticholinergics
        phenytoin
        barbiturates
        digoxin
        levadopa
    miscellaneous
        constipation
        urinary retention
        intraabdominal pathology e.g. sepsis, mesenteric infarction
        arteritis

Clinical features
　　clouding of consciousness leading to impairment of mental
　　　　clarity
　　disorientation in time, place and person
　　agitation
　　hallucinations may be present
　　incontinence

Treatment
　　treat the underlying cause
　　for agitation and confusion
　　　　thioridazine 10 mg t.d.s., or haloperidol 0.5 mg b.d. or t.d.s.,
　　　　　　or chlorpromazine 50–100 mg oral or i.m. repeated until
　　　　　　sedation obtained
　　　　for severe toxic confusion i.v. infusion of chlormethiazole
　　　　　　may be used

Constipation

Aetiology
> low intake of food (fibre)
> immobility
> colonic lesions
>> diverticular disease
>> carcinoma
>> bowel atonia
>> 'cathartic' colon
>> idiopathic megacolon
> anal – painful lesions
>> fissure
>> abscess
>> haemorrhoids
> metabolic
>> myxoedema
>> hypokalaemia
>> hypercalcaemia
>> dehydration
>> porphyria
> drugs
>> codeine
>> tricyclic antidepressants
>> laxative (dependance)
>> anti-hypertensives
>> anti-cholinergics
> miscellaneous
>> depression
>> Parkinson's disease
>> CVA
>> pelvic tumour

Complications
> **impaction with faecal incontinence**
> **urinary retention with overflow incontinence**
> **confusion**

Treatment
> treat the underlying cause
> purgatives
>> bulk producers – bran, methylcellulose (1–1.5 g in the morning)
>> stimulants – senna (5–10 mg nocte)

osmotic agents – lactulose (10–15 ml daily according to response)

lubricants – liquid paraffin (15–45 ml in the evening)

for severe constipation with impaction enemas and manual removal may have to be tried

Deep Vein Thrombosis

Aetiology
immobility
± other factors
dehydration
diuretic therapy
polycythaemia
thrombocytosis
dysproteinaemias
neoplasia
obstruction of pelvic veins

Clinical features
oedema of lower leg
calf tenderness
pyrexia
confusion
Homan's sign not useful in elderly
complications
pulmonary embolism
leg ulceration
long-standing oedema

Investigations – if available – use
venography
ultrasound, or
[^{125}I]fibrinogen uptake

Treatment
elevation of leg
compression bandage
analgesics for pain
anticoagulants
heparin 10 000 units six hourly or 30–40 000 units in 50 ml
given over 24 hours using an infusion pump + warfarin
20–25 mg as a loading dose. After 48 hours warfarin
dose calculated according to prothrombin time and
heparin stopped after 36 hours
NB special precautions:-
recent stroke
history of peptic ulcer
history of hiatus hernia
liver disease
congestive heart failure

NB contraindications:
    recent cerebral haemorrhage
    active gastrointestinal bleeding
    bleeding diathesis
    severe hypertension

Depression

Incidence: 8–15% in general population

Commonest mental illness in the elderly

Aetiology
- **loss of health**
- **loss of work role**
- **financial worrying**
- **loss of spouse**
- **social isolation**
- **incontinence**
- secondary to any severe ilness
    - **carcinoma**
    - **myxoedema**
    - **thyrotoxicosis**
    - **Parkinson's disease**
    - **drugs**
        - antihypertensives
            - methyldopa
            - propranolol
            - reserpine
        - anti-parkinsonian drugs
            - levadopa
            - bromocriptine
        - antidepressants
            - amitriptyline
            - doxepin
        - corticosteroids
        - phenothiazines
        - barbiturates
        - digitalis

Clinical features
- typical presentation
    - anorexia
    - weight loss
    - memory loss
    - increasing frailty
    - apathy
    - constipation
    - multiple somatic complaints
- atypical presentation
    - hypochondriasis – fear of cancer etc.

'pseudodementia'
>poor concentration
>poor recall
>disorientation
>
>severe localized pain
>
>alcohol or drug addiction – rare presentation of depression
>
suicide common

Treatment
>psychotherapy +
>
>tricyclic or tetracyclic antidepressants
>
>tricyclics
>>imipramine 10–25 mg t.d.s.
>>
>>amitriptyline 10 mg t.d.s. (for those who need sedation also)
>>
>>amitriptyline 25–50 mg nocte if side effects like drowsiness and hypotension during day-time are severe
>>
>>if response to tricyclics not adequate check serum levels since poor response can occur with very low or very high levels
>>
>>**side effects of tricyclics**
>>>blurring of vision
>>>retention of urine
>>>postural hypotension
>>>cardiac arrhythmias
>>>confusion
>
>tetracyclic – maprotiline hydrochloride 25–150 mg daily in divided doses
>
>other antidepressants (apart from tricyclics or tetracyclics) – L-tryptophan 1–2 g t.d.s. – main side-effect is drowsiness
>
>ECT used for severe depression – main side effect of this is short-term memory loss

Diabetes Mellitus

Random blood sugar >10 mmol/l
Two-hour post 50 g of glucose: 8–10 mmol/l
Two types
    juvenile – severe, insulin eventually required

    maturity onset
        mild
        usually controlled by diet ± hypoglycaemic agents
        insulin only occasionally required

Clinical features of presentation
    classical symptoms (polyuria, polydypsia, weight loss etc.), or
        incidental finding of glycosuria or hyperglycaemia, or complications
        cataract
        retinopathy (microaneurysms, haemorrhages, exudates)
        peripheral neuropathy
        autonomic neuropathy
        nephropathy – presenting initially with proteinuria only
        myocardial infarction (common cause of death in diabetics)
        peripheral vascular disease
        foot ulceration
        coma
            hypoglycaemia
            hyperglycaemic ketoacidosis
            non-ketotic hyperosmolar – precipitated by thiazides, carbohydrate drinks
            lactic acidosis
                (phenformin-taking diabetic
               induced by precipitating factors like myocardial infarction, renal failure etc.
               high mortality
               treatment – large amounts of bicarbonate)
Treatment
    diet – 100–150 g of carbohydrate diet usually sufficient
    drugs
        sulphonylureas
            stimulate secretion of insulin
            tolbutamide (500–1500 mg/day) is the drug of choice as it has short half life
            chlorpropamide not indicated in elderly – risk of hypoglycaemia very high with this long acting agent

biguanides
> metformin - usually only added if diabetes is difficult to control on maximum dosage of tolbutamide and patient is unlikely or reluctant to take insulin

insulin
> if treatment with oral agents fail
>
> if patient goes into hyperglycaemic coma

foot care - regular visit to chiropodist essential

regular ophthalmic supervision to detect
> cataract
>
> proliferative retinopathy as it is treatable by photocoagulation

Epilepsy

Definition: abnormal paroxysmal electrical cerebral discharge

Types
    focal
    generalized (grand mal)
    temporal lobe

Aetiology
    cerebrovascular disease – commonest
    tumour: primary or secondary cerebral tumour
    cerebral anoxia e.g. cardiac dysrrhythmias
    trauma
        post-traumatic
        subdural haematoma
    subarachnoid haemorrhage
    metabolic
        respiratory failure
        renal failure
        hepatic failure
        hypoglycaemia
        hypocalcaemia
        water intoxication
    infections
        viral or bacterial (meningitis, encephalitis)
        abscess
    drugs
        barbiturate withdrawal
        chlorpromazine
        amitriptyline
        lignocaine
        respiratory stimulants

Treatment
    phenytoin
        50–150 mg/day
        dose can be monitored using blood levels
        side-effects: ataxia, nystagmus, macrocytic anaemia, hir-
           sutes, gum hypertrophy
    primidone 250 mg t.d.s. or q.d.s.
    sodium valporate – start with 200 mg t.d.s. – usual maintenance
        1–1.6 g /day

phenobarbitone
> **if possible should be avoided in the elderly – risk of osteomalacia and dementia high with use of barbiturates in the elderly**

carbamazepine for focal or temporal lobe fits

in emergency use diazepam IV

Fractures

Aetiology
    fall ±
        osteoporosis
        osteomalacia
        Paget's disease
        malignancy
        bone cysts
        steroids etc.

Types
    femur
        commonest type of fracture
        affects 2% of women and 1% of men aged 85 and over
          annually
        neck
            subcapital
            pertrochanteric
        clinical features
            pain
            externally rotated leg
            immobility
            if impacted – pain and shortening only, patient can be
              mobile
        treatment
            internal fixation, or prosthesis e.g. Thompson's
              prosthesis, + rehabilitation post-surgery
    humerus
        most impacted
        treatment
            collar and cuff sling
            if not impacted internal fixation
  Colle's fracture – treatment: manipulation and plaster backslab
  pelvic fractures: treatment symptomatic
        if unstable internal fixation
  fracture near ankle: treatment – plaster
        if ankle joint involved internal fixation
  fracture in foot: treatment – compression bandage
  fracture of trunk
    compression fracture
    treatment
        symptomatic (pain relief)
        corset

rib fractures: treatment symptomatic (pain relief)
        if flail chest present tight strapping necessary
pathological fractures – require internal fixation + radiotherapy
  or chemotherapy
general effects of fractures
    confusion
    in case of fractures in legs
        immobility
        bed sores
        incontinence
        thromboembolism
        wound infection after operation

Fungal Infections

Candida

involves mouth, vulva, groin, perianal, submammary etc.

common in
> **bedridden patients**
> **patients with malignant disease**
> **patients on steroids or cytotoxic agents or antibiotics**
> **diabetics**

treatment
> nystatin pessaries for vaginal candida
> nystatin suspension for oral candida infection
> amphotericin lozenges if nystatin not available

Cryptococcus

seen in debilitated immunoparetic patients or in malignancy
systemic infection
meningitis
usually fatal
diagnosed by
> staining sputum or CSF with india ink
> culture

treatment
> amphotericin B – 1–5 mg in 5% dextrose given over six hours: injections repeated on alternate days until 3 g has been given
> 5-fluorcytosine 100–200 $mg\,kg^{-1}\,day^{-1}$

Aspergillus fumigatus

aspergilloma (occuring in lung cavity or bulla), or
aspergillosis, or
pulmonary eosinophilia related to exposure
clinical features
> asymptomatic, or
> pneumonia, or
> acute asthma with eosinophilia

diagnosis
> precipitin test +ve
> radiology

treatment
> resection for localized aspergilloma
> amphotericin B
> steroids for asthma

Ringworm of feet
>	types
>>		*Trichophyton mentagrophytes*
>>		*Trichophyton robrum*
>>		*Epidermophyton fluccosum*

Ringworm of scalp
>	*Microsporum audouini*
>	*Microsporum canis*
>	treatment
>>		griseofulvin 125 mg q.d.s. for about one month
>>		Whitfield's ointment

Gall Stones

Incidence
about 15–20%
increases with age

Types
pure cholesterol
pure pigment
mixed

Factors associated
infection
increased saturation of bile
bile stasis
drugs e.g. clofibrate, cholestyramine
chronic haemolysis
terminal ileal disease

Clinical features
often asymptomatic (50%) especially in the elderly
cholecystitis associated with pain, fever, jaundice and confusion
obstructive jaundice
gall stone ileus
particularly common in elderly women
stone lodges at terminal ileum usually but occasionally it
can lodge in duodenum or jejunum
mortality well over 30%
signs and symptoms of pancreatitis
empyema of gall bladder
carcinoma of gall bladder

Investigations
plain abdomen – may show radio-opaque stones
cholecystogram
performed usually after an acute attack of cholecystitis has
settled
may show non-functioning gall bladder or presence of gall
stones
ultrasound – can show up gall stones as well as size of gall
bladder

Treatment
if silent – none
if symptoms present
cholecystitis: analgesia, fluids IV, and antibiotics

pure cholesterol stones (<10 mm in diameter):
  chenodeoxycholic acid 10–15 mg kg^{-1} day^{-1}
  contraindicated in patients with liver disease
surgery for
  recurrent cholecystitis
  obstructive jaundice
  some cases of gall stone ileus
  empyema of gall bladder

Giant Cell Arteritis

Definition: vasculitis involving large or medium sized arteries

Aetiology – not known

Clinical features
    male:female ratio equal
    headache:scalp tenderness frequent
    fever
    malaise
    fatigue
    weight loss – may precede headache
    tender, palpable temporal arteries
    muscle pain, stiffness and weakness (may present as poly-
        myalgia rheumatica)
    visual failure (retinal artery thrombosis)
    stroke
    'pulseless disease' – if aortic arch involved
    pain in face or jaw (occasionally 'claudication' of muscles of
        mastication)

Investigation
    ESR high although can be normal
    normochromic, normocytic anaemia
    temporal artery biopsy: diagnostic changes if affected area
        selected
    chronic inflammatory changes with accumulation of lympho-
        cytes, macrophages, plasma cells and giant cells. **Changes**
        may be segmental

Treatment
    systemic steroids
    prednisone 60 mg per day – reducing rapidly to maintenance
        level, aiming to keep ESR in normal range

Glaucoma

Intraocular pressure > 21 mmHg
Accounts for 13% of those registered as blind

Acute closed angle glaucoma
(increased intraocular pressure from blockage of angle of anterior chamber by iris)
clinical features
painful red eye
transient blurring of vision
rainbow-coloured 'haloes' (often precipitated at first by poor lighting or emotion)
semi-dilated oval pupil
headache
nausea and vomiting
often in hypermetropic eyes (rare in myopia)

treatment
pilocarpine 4% drops every 5 minutes for ½ hour, every ½ hour for 2 hours, then q.d.s.
acetazolamide 500 mg orally, then 250 mg q.d.s.
occasionally oral glycerol or 20% mannitol i.v.
subsequently, peripheral iridectomy or drainage procedure

Chronic open angle glaucoma
primary
secondary to
uveitis
retinal vein thrombosis
diabetes etc.
clinical features
usually initially asymptomatic
may present with visual loss from optic nerve damage – nasal field initially affected and often unnoticed
optic cupping on fundoscopy
treatment
pilocarpine ½–4% q.d.s. or other miotic drops
β-blockers can also be used to lower ocular pressure
surgery
anterior sclerectomy
trabeculectomy

Hazards of Drugs

Problems caused by
    incorrect therapy
    inadquate supervision
    failure to give adequate information to patient
    failure of patient to follow instructions – non-compliance –
        due to
            poor vision
            deafness
            dementia etc.
    poly-pharmacy
    altered drug metabolism
        fall in renal function
        fall in carrier proteins
        .˙. distribution and metabolism of drugs is affected
        fall in hepatic function e.g oxidation
    increased sensitivity to drugs with age – elderly are more
        prone to side-effects

Common side-effects produced by drugs
    confusion
            amitrityline
            anticholinergics
            analgesics
            sedatives
            digoxin
            isoniazid
            levadopa
    hallucinations
            levadopa
            amitriptyline
            amantadine
            methyldopa
            prednisone
            propranolol
            metronidazole
    convulsions
            chlorpromazine
            imipramine
            amitriptyline
    extrapyramidal syndromes
            chlorpromazine
            haloperidol

levadopa
imipramine
thioridazine
metoclopramide
flaccid weakness
steroids
diphenylhydantoins
sulphonamides
tetracyclines
neomycin
phenothiazines
carbenoxolone
procainamide
peripheral neuropathy
nitrofurantoin
amitrityline
imipramine
hydralazine
phenylbutazone
carbamazepine
perhexilene
nystagmus
barbiturates
diphenylhydantoins
meprobamate
chlordiazepoxide
depression
methyldopa
propranolol
reserpine
levadopa
bromocriptine
steroids
barbiturates
digoxin
amitriptyline
doxepin
pulmonary oedema
carbenoxolone
phenylbutazone
propranolol
salicylates

        steroids
        cardiodepressants e.g. verapamil, nifidipine, perhexilene etc.
pulmonary eosinophilia
        penicillin
        nitrofurantoin
        isoniazid
        sulphonamides
        PAS
lipoid pneumonia
        liquid paraffin
nausea and vomiting
        digoxin
        levadopa
        bromocriptine
        analgesics
        stilboestrol etc.
constipation
        ganglion blocking drugs
        opiates etc.
        tricyclic antidepressants (adynamic ileus) etc.
bleeding from gastrointestinal tract
        salicylates
        steroids
        phenylbutazone
        indomethacin
        digitalis
        potassium salts
megaloblastic anaemia
        methotrexate
        nitrofurantoin
        phenylbutazone
        phenytoin
        primidone
haemolytic anaemia
        methyldopa
        isoniazid
        chloramphenicol
        nalidixic acid
        penicillin (high dose)
        quinine
aplastic anaemia
        chloramphenicol

chlorpromazine
chlorthiazide
chlorpropamide
tolbutamide
aspirin
carbamazine, sulphonamides etc.

jaundice
    hepatocellular
        tetracycline
        methyldopa
        isoniazid
        nitrofurantoin
        benzodiazepines
    cholestatic
        phenothiazines
        methyltestosterone
        chlorpropamide
        erythromycin
        rifampicin
    mixed
        phenytoin
Stevens–Johnson syndrome
    barbiturates
    sulphonamides
    phenylbutazone
    phenytoin
lymphadenopathy
    barbiturates
    salicylates
    nalidixic acid
    phenytoin

Interaction of commonly used drugs
    anticoagulants
        activity reduced
            barbiturates
            phenytoin
            carbamazepine
        activity increased
            salicylates
            alcohol
            clofibrate

thiouracils
broad spectrum antibiotics
sulphonylureas

tolbutamide
    activity increased
        dicoumarol
        chloramphenicol
        phenylbutazone
        propranolol
        steroids
        sulphonamides
    activity reduced
        thiazide diuretics

phenytoin
    activity increased
        isoniazid
        chloramphenicol
        dicoumarol
        phenylbutazone

penicillin
    activity increased
        probenecid

cephalothin
    activity increased
        probenecid

antihypertensive drugs
    activity increased
        sedatives
        antidepressants
        narcotic analgesics
        phenothiazines

levadopa
    activity reduced
        methyldopa
        haloperidol
        phenothiazines

Heart Failure

Aetiology
  ischaemic heart disease (commonest) + precipitating factor(s)
      chest infection
      myocardial infarction
      arrhythmias
      pulmonary embolic disease
      anaemia
      thyrotoxicosis
      drugs (producing hypotension or arrhythmia)
  hypertensive heart disease
  cardiomyopathy
      amyloid
      thyrotoxicosis
      myxoedema
      sarcoidosis
      beriberi
  constrictive pericarditis
      idiopathic
      tuberculosis
      post-pyogenic e.g. staphylococcal
      malignancy
  pericardial effusion
      malignancy
      myxoedema
      anticoagulants – if used when pericarditis is present
  valvular disease ± bacterial endocarditis
  cor pulmonale
      acute or chronic
      secondary to chronic lung disease, pulmonary embolic
          disease
  miscellaneous
      Paget's disease
      anaemia

Clinical features
  left ventricular failure
      breathlessness
      orthopnoea
      paroxysmal nocturnal dyspnoea
      bilateral basal crepitations
  right ventricular failure
      oedema
      hepatomegaly

JVP↑
tachycardia
pleural effusions and ascites occasionally present in
    severe failure
third and fourth sounds

Treatment
    diuretics
            frusemide or bumetanide with potassium supplements or
            ethacrynic acid for acute attack
            for maintenance therapy – a mild diuretic (thiazide) with
            potassium or combination of spironolactone with
            thiazide may be used
    digoxin – if fast fibrillation is present
    oxygen and opiates in acute left ventricular failure

Hiatus Hernia

Two types
> sliding: oesophago-gastric junction moves up through the diaphragmatic hiatus into chest – most common type
> rolling: fundus of stomach herniates through the hiatus

Clinical features
> usually that of oesophageal reflux
> substernal pain
> dysphagia
> acid reflux in mouth
> frequency 10–30%
> complications
>> oesophagitis
>> oesophageal stricture
>> anaemia from bleeding – 10–40% patients with hiatus hernia are anaemic
>> **aspiration leading to cough and diffuse pulmonary fibrosis – more common in the elderly**
> diagnosis made on
>> clinical history
>> barium swallow with head down view or on endoscopy

Treatment
> avoid stooping
> avoid constricting garments
> sleep propped up
> stop smoking
> drugs
>> antacids for symptomatic relief of oesophageal reflux
>> gaviscon (alginic acid and antacid mixture) – a surface acting agent
>> metoclopramide hydrochloride 5–10 mg t.d.s. to increase the tone of the lower oesophageal sphincter
>> for oesophagitis or peptic ulcer: use cimetidine 200 mg t.d.s. and 400 mg at night or 'pyrogastrone', a mixture containing carbenoxolone
> surgery
>> for those with persistence of oesophagitis despite medical treatment
>> for recurrent bleeding
>> for stricture
>> **NB repair operation is not always successful**

Hypercalcaemia

Serum calcium >2.59 mmol/l for men and >2.68 mmol/l for women

Aetiology
> **neoplasm with or without metastases**
> myelomatosis
> vitamin D intoxication
> milk alkali syndrome (Burnett's syndrome)
> hyperparathyroidism – primary or tertiary
> thyrotoxicosis (rare)
> **Paget's disease (+ immobilization)**
> sarcoidosis (hypersensitivity to vitamin D – usually with severe
> disease)

Clinical features
> anorexia
> nausea
> vomiting
> **constipation**
> dyspepsia (+ peptic ulceration with 1° hyperparathyroidism)
> polyuria
> polydypsia
> fatigue
> **depression**
> psychosis
> **dementia**
> renal stone formation
> nephrocalcinosis
> band keratopathy: calcification in cornea at limbus may be seen
> in hyperparathyroidism
> bone disease with hyperparathyroidism
> > osteitis fibrosa cystica
> > subperiosteal resorption of phalanges

Treatment
> rehydration
> frusemide after rehydration
> treat underlying disorder
> vitamin D – withdraw/reduce dose
> milk alkali – substitute non-absorbable alkali
> steroids – except in hyperparathyroidism
> sarcoidosis – avoid sunlight
> treat malignancy – chemotherapy if disseminated – local treat-
> ment if appropriate
> mobilization/calcitonin for Paget's disease

surgery for parathyroid tumour
In emergency
    (1) rehydrate ⎤
       frusemide ⎦
    (2) phosphate infusion may be necessary occasionally if
       patient unconscious and does not respond to (1). NB
       metastatic calcification will occur

Hypertension

Definition: BP > 200/110 mmHg in elderly
Affects about 15% of population

Aetiology
    essential
    renal disease
        chronic pyelonephritis
        analgesic nephropathy
        diabetic renal disease
        renal ischaemia
        glomerulonephritis
    adrenal disease
        Conn's syndrome (primary hyperaldosteronism)
        Cushing's disease – rare
    drugs
        steroids
        oestrogens
        carbenoxolone

Clinical features
    asymptomatic
    left ventricular hypertrophy
    angina
    heart failure
    fundal changes
        AV nipping and silver wiring of arteries common but
        haemorrhages, exudates and papilloedema (changes
        of malignant hypertension) rare in the elderly
    complications
        stroke
        myocardial infarction
        subarachnoid haemorrhage
        dissecting aneurysm
        renal failure
        peripheral vascular disease

Treatment
    given only if hypertension sustained or symptoms present –
    aim for BP of 180/100
    drugs
        diuretics – thiazide with potassium supplements or a
        combination of thiazide and spironolactone

NB side-effects of thiazide are
   potassium depletion
   hyperglycaemia
   hyperuricaemia
   thrombocytopenic purpura
beta-adrenergic blockers
   propranolol 120–240 mg/day depending on pulse
      rate
   oxprenolol 160–320 mg/day
hydrallazine
   used if thiazide and/or beta-adrenergic blockers fail
      to control BP or if patient can not tolerate them
   25 mg b.d. or t.d.s. to maximum of 200 mg/day
methyldopa
   another alternative to treatment
   125–750 mg/day in divided doses is usually suf-
      ficient in most patients
   NB side-effects
      depression
      lassitude
      postural hypotension
      +ve Coomb's test – 10–30% have this but
         haemolytic anaemia with symptoms is rare

Hypocalcaemia

Serum calcium < 2.18 mmol/l

Aetiology
> **hypoalbuminaemia – common cause of spurious low calcium
> in the elderly**
> vitamin D deficiency
> hypoparathyroidism
>> primary
>> secondary to thyroid surgery, parathyroid surgery
> renal failure
> steatorrhoea

Clinical features
> paresthesiae
> tetany
> convulsions
> Trousseau's sign +ve
> Chvostek's +ve
> depression
> psychotic behaviour
> cataract
> atrophy of nails
> monilial infection
> chronic hypocalcaemia leads to brain calcification, especially
> basal ganglia

Treatment
> if symptoms present – calcium gluconate (10%) 20 ml i.v.
> calciferol (1.25–2.5 mg/day) or 1,a-hydroxycholecalciferol in
> case of hypoparathyroidism, renal failure or steatorrhoea.
> With this treatment serum calcium has to be monitored
> carefully

Hypokalaemia

Serum potassium < 3.5 mmol/l

Aetiology
    inadequate intake – poor diet (poverty, isolation, immobility)
    loss from gut
        vomiting
        diarrhoea
            ulcerative colitis
            purgative abuse
            villous adenoma
            fistulae
            steatorrhoea
    loss from kidney
        recovery from obstruction
        renal tubular acidosis
        diuretics
    metabolic causes
        Cushing's disease
        aldosteronism
        keto-acidosis
    drugs
        diuretics
        steroids
        carbenoxolone

Clinical features
    weakness
    immobility
    confusion
    abdominal distension (paralytic ileus)
    cardiac arrhythmias
    ECG changes
        flat T wave
        U wave
    rarely tetany

Treatment
    increase dietary intake e.g. fruit
    potassium supplements

Hyponatraemia

Plasma sodium < 132 mmol/l

Aetiology
(1) loss of sodium without proportionate loss of water:
  loss from gut
    vomiting
    diarrhoea including purgatives
    small bowel obstruction
  loss from kidney
    renal tubular defect – e.g. post obstruction, tubular necrosis etc.
    diabetic ketoacidosis
    diuretics
  Addison's disease
(2) retention of water without proportionate retention of sodium
  inappropriate ADH:
    malignancy (especially oat cell bronchogenic carcinoma)
    respiratory infection
    trauma
    tuberculosis
    myxoedema
    chlorpropamide
(3) loss of cellular homeostatic mechanisms
    severe general illness – 'sick cell syndrome'

Clinical features
  asymptomatic until $Na^+ < 120$ mmol/l
  'water intoxication'
    confusion
    irritability
    convulsions
    coma

Treatment
(1) sodium loss: replacement therapy
(2) inappropriate ADH secretion
    restrict fluids
    demeclo-cycline or chlortetracycline
    hypertonic saline in emergency

Hypothermia

Definition: rectal temperature $< 35°C$

Aetiology:
- **exposure to low ambient temperature (inadequate clothing, inadequate heating, open windows etc.)**
- **defective thermoregulatory mechanism ±**
  - **fall**
  - **stroke**
  - **myxoedema** (decreased metabolism)
  - **drugs**
    - phenothiazines
    - barbiturates
    - alcohol
  - **intellectual failure**

Clinical features
- low core temperature
- may have cold extremities
- pale skin
- puffy face (resembles myxoedematous facies)
- slow respiration
- slow pulse rate – sinus bradycardia
- may have slurred speech, muscle rigidity or flap
- extensor planters
- 'J' waves on ECG
- **reflexes may show slow relaxation phase without the presence of myxoedema**
- **complications**
  - **gastric dilatation – common, risk of aspiration high**
  - acute pancreatitis – often asymptomatic
  - bronchopneumonia
  - cardiac arrhythmias
    - supraventricular tachycardia
    - atrial fibrillation
    - ventricular tachycardia
    - ventricular fibrillation
    - heart block, etc.
  - thromboembolism
  - death

Treatment
- **slow rewarming using space blanket (0.5°C per hour) – rapid rewarming may lead to cardiac arrhythmias**

cardiac monitoring to detect and treat arrhythmias
antibiotics e.g. ampicillin for chest infection
fluids if dehydration present
tri-iodothyronine if myxoedema present
hydrocortisone in very ill patient although its value is debatable
gastric tube for aspiration if gastric dilatation suspected

cf. Heat stroke

Aetiology
high environmental temperature (heat wave) +
impaired thermoregulatory mechanism – diminished or absent
sweating

Clinical features
high rectal temperature (average above 41°C)
dehydration with no sweating
coma
prodromally some patients may have
nausea
vomiting
anorexia
weakness
dyspnoea
dizziness
feeling hot
serum chloride high
serum sodium high
bronchopneumonia common
mortality high

Treatment
cooling with sponges
i.v. fluids
antibiotics if bronchopneumonia present

Hypothyroidism

Accounts for 3-5% of all admissions to geriatric hospital

Aetiology
    primary
        autoimmune thyroiditis
    secondary
        hypopituitarism
        following thyroid surgery or iodine–131 treatment for thyrotoxicosis

Clinical features
    insidious onset in the elderly who are usually females
    physical and mental slowness
    depression
    constipation
    weakness
    impaired mobility
    intolerance to cold
    hoarseness of voice
    cold dry coarse skin
    hair loss
    dementia
    slow relaxation of reflexes
    rarely patient may present with
        neuropathy
        hypothermia
        myxoedema coma
        carpal tunnel syndrome
        pericardial effusion
        ascites
        cerebellar ataxia

Investigations
    $T_4\downarrow$
    $T_3\downarrow$ (NB T_3 tends to fall with age)
    $\uparrow$TSH in primary thyroid failure
    ECG
        low voltage complexes
        bradycardia
        flattened T wave etc.
    blood film – $1/3$ have anaemia – normochromic normocytic or macrocytic – this improves with treatment

Treatment
thyroxine – start with 50 μg/day, increase by 50 μg at weekly intervals to maintenance dose of 150–200 μg/day
tri-iodothyronine 10–20 μg 12-hourly is used in myxoedema coma

Immobility

Any illness causing an elderly person to go to bed is likely to lead to immobility.

Specific causes
 neurological
   cerebrovascular accident
   transient ischaemic attacks
   Parkinson's disease
   disseminated sclerosis
   encephalitis
   motor neurone disease
   peripheral neuropathy
   cord lesions
   cauda equina lesions
   Alzheimer's disease (late)
 musculoskeletal
   arthritis (see p. 51)
   polymyositis
   myasthaenia gravis
   Paget's disease of bone
   osteomalacia
   fractures (especially femoral)
   any disorder causing muscular wasting
   pain in legs
   pain in back (see p. 30)
 metabolic
   hypokalaemia
   myxoedema
   Cushing's disease
   thyrotoxicosis (apathetic form or myopathy)
 drugs
   sedatives
   hypotensives
   phenothiazines
   carbenoxolone
   steroids etc.
 miscellaneous
   depression
   recurrent falls from any cause (see p. 18) giving rise to loss of confidence

Common complications
    pressure sores
    osteoporosis
    hypostatic pneumonia
    hypothermia
    muscular contractures

Treatment
    of underlying cause if possible
    physiotherapy

    **NB For elderly patients, early identification of susceptible
    subjects is important: recognition and treatment of dis-
    orders likely to produce immobility: prevention of recur-
    rence, if necessary by continuing therapy in Day Hospital**

117

Incontinence (urinary)

Definition: (by Brocklehurst) incontinence is present if the answer to the question 'Does urine ever come away unexpectedly and without your being able to stop it and you get wet?' is 'yes'.

Incidence: 20-30%

Aetiology
    treatable
        infection
        pelvis SOL especially faeces
        senile vaginitis
        immobility
        diuretic therapy
        diabetes mellitus
        hypercalcaemia
        prostatic hypertrophy
        bladder calculi
        cystocoele
        stress incontinence
    partially treatable
        carcinoma of bladder
        loss of cortical inhibition (cerebrovascular disease, tumour etc.)
        unstable bladder (bladder dyssynergia)
    untreatable
        cauda equina lesions (trauma, tumour etc.)
        posterior nerve root lesions (tabes dorsalis, diabetes mellitus)
        loss of afferent and efferent fibres
            road traffic accident
            post-rectal surgery

Treatment
        treat infection if present
        treat constipation if present
        for vaginitis – local or oral oestrogens (quinestradiol 500 μg b.d.)
        for stress incontinence
            physiotherapy
            surgery to elevate bladder neck

for unstable or uninhibited bladder use anticholinergics
empronium hydrochloride 200–400 mg nocte
for day-time incontinence 200 mg t.d.s. can be tried
flavoxate two tabs t.d.s.
for untreatable incontinence use aids available: incontinence pads, kanga pants, catheter etc.

Infective Endocarditis

Aetiology
>   *Streptococcus viridans* – commonest
>   *Streptococcus faecalis*
>   *Staphylococcus, streptococcus pneumoniae*
>   *E. coli*
>   less common organisms in debilitated or immunoparetic patients or those with prosthetic heart valves

Source of infection
>   infected skin lesions
>   dental manipulation
>   **bladder (catheterization)**

Pathology
>   organism may infect a valve previously damaged by any process
>   **commonly sclerotic aortic valve in elderly**
>   highly pathogenic organism may attack a previously normal valve

Clinical features
>   **general ill health**
>   **weight loss**
>   low grade fever
>   **confusion**
>   atrial fibrillation
>   heart block (vegetation involving conducting tissue)
>   congestive cardiac failure
>   **murmur – changing murmur uncommon feature in elderly**
>   systemic emboli

>   finger clubbing – late feature
>   immune complexes – glomerular disease – microscopic haematuria – Osler's nodes (finger palps) – splinter haemorrhages (nails) – 'Roth spots' (fundi), Janeway spots (hands)
>   NB features of septicaemia in presence of more virulent organism

Investigation
>   blood cultures (not less than three) – 10–30% have sterile cultures
>   anaemia (normochromic normocytic)
>   ESR raised
>   haematuria (microscopic)
>   immune complexes
>   specific antibodies to rare pathogens – e.g. *Candida,* Q fever

Treatment

penicillin and streptomycin until organism and its sensitivity known

penicillin 6–12 mega-units per day parenterally

streptomycin 0.75 g i.m. b.d. Agent used subsequently depends on blood cultures

dose subsequently depends on bacteriocidal levels achieved in the serum

duration of therapy ranges from 4 to 6 weeks, but may be longer

valve replacement may be necessary if eradication of organism is not achieved or if serious haemodynamic problems result due to valvular incompetence or in the case of infected prosthetic valves

Prophylactic antibiotics

used when valvular disease is present for all dental manipulation and genito-urinary procedures

the agent used depending on likely organism present

for dental procedures: penicillin 1 mega-unit parenterally ½ hour before and Pen V 500 mg q.d.s. for 48 hours

for genito-urinary procedures: ampicillin 500 mg parenterally ½ hour preceding and 250 mg q.d.s. for 48 hours

Intracranial Tumours

Types
>gliomas
>**meningioma – commonest**
>acoustic neuroma
>pituitary tumours
>secondary deposits – from carcinoma of
>>lung (accounts for 30–40% of all cerebral secondaries)
>>stomach
>>breast
>>kidney etc.

Clinical features
>localizing symptoms
>>weakness
>>hemianopia
>>diplopia etc.
>non-localizing
>>headache
>>epilepsy
>>confusion etc.
>false localizing
>>due to raised intracranial pressure
>>sixth nerve palsy
>>cerebellar signs
>>extrapyramidal syndromes
>**papilloedema commonly seen in younger group with cerebral tumours is rare in the elderly**
>**(NB non-metastatic neurological complications of tumours, e.g.**
>>**dementia**
>>**peripheral neuropathy**
>>**myasthenic syndrome**
>>**cerebellar degeneration etc.)**

Investigations
>skull X-rays
>>in some pineal shift may be seen
>>in case of meningioma a local erosion or a thickening of bone may be seen
>isotopic brain scan – increased uptake seen in the region of tumour

computer-assisted tomography
   investigation of choice
   allows good anatomical localization
   often helps with aetiology

Treatment
   benign tumours like meningiomas may be resected
   malignant tumours (primary or secondary)
      radiotherapy to give short-term symptomatic relief may be
         tried
      steroids may also be used to reduce intracranial pressure
         and thus improve symptoms on short-term basis

Ischaemic Heart Disease

Coronary heart disease accounts for over $1/3$ deaths in elderly

Risk factors
 hyperlipidaemia – particularly ↑ cholesterol and ↑ low density or
  very low density lipoprotein
 (factors associated with hyperlipidaemia are
   hereditary
   diet
   diabetes mellitus
   hypothyroidism
   alcohol ingestion
   hyperuricaemia)
 diabetes mellitus
 hypertension
 cigarette smoking
 obesity
 inactivity

Presentations
 asymptomatic
 angina
   central chest pain related to effort or emotion
   breathlessness
   discomfort in chest on exertion
   examination usually normal but during attack 4th heart
    sound may be heard

   treatment
     glyceryl trinitrate sublingually
     for prophylaxis
       beta-adrenergic blockers
       nifidipine
       perhexilene
     oral diuretics may help nocturnal angina
 myocardial infarction
   chest pain (heavy, crushing, tightness)
     can be absent in elderly
   dyspnoea
   hypotension
     acute confusional state
   dizziness
   syncope
   fall

complications
    arrhythmias
    shock
    septal perforation
    papillary muscle rupture
    venous or arterial thrombosis
    arterial emboli
    Dressler's syndrome
    shoulder - hand syndrome
    stroke
ECG
    can be normal
    may show typical changes of infarct e.g. q wave with raised ST segment
enzymes
    SGOT and CPK raised early after myocardial infarction and fall to normal in 3 days
    HBD rises during 1st day, has peak at 3–4th day and returns to normal in 14 days
arrhythmias – see p. 61

Malabsorption

Aetiology
    stomach
        post-gastrectomy
        post-vagotomy
        (atrophic gastritis)
    intestine
        resection or bypass operation
        coeliac disease
        tropical sprue
        intestinal ischaemia
        jejunal diverticuli
        strictures
        enteritis e.g. *Salmonella*
        parasitic infestation e.g. *Giardia*
        lymphoma
        Whipple's disease
    pancreas
        chronic pancreatitis
        tumour of head of pancreas
        Zollinger–Ellison syndrome
    liver
        obstructive jaundice
        parenchymal liver disease
    cardiovascular
        constrictive pericarditis
        congestive heart failure
        vasculitis
    metabolic
        thyrotoxicosis
        hypoparathyroidism
        diabetes mellitus
        carcinoid syndrome
    drugs
        neomycin
        PAS
        phenindione
        cholestyramine
        antibiotics
    miscellaneous
        widespread skin disease
        scleroderma
        idiopathic

Clinical features
    diarrhoea
    steatorrhoea
    weight loss
    anorexia
    weakness
    nutritional deficiencies with complications e.g. osteomalacia

Investigations
    depend on suspected cause
    5 day faecal fat
    xylose absorption test – oral and intravenous
    isotopic [^{14}C]glycocholate breath test – if bacterial overgrowth
        suspected
    small bowel biopsy – useful in suspected coeliac disease,
        amyloid, lymphoma etc.
    barium meal and follow through – shows flocculation and
        clumping of barium in malabsorption
    culture of stools and search for parasites
    pancreatic function
            endoscopic retrograde cannulation of pancreas useful in
                diagnosis of suspected pancreatic disease
            ultrasound
    5HIAA for carcinoid +
    nutritional screen

Treatment
    depends on cause
    replacement of nutritional deficiencies

Motor Neurone Disease

Definition: degeneration of anterior horn cells in spinal cord and in motor cranial nuclei and pyramidal tracts

Incidence: 1 per 100 000 per year

Prevalence: 2.5–7 per 100 000

Clinical forms
- amyotrophic lateral sclerosis
    - upper motor neurone signs
    - weakness
    - spasticity
    - hyperreflexia
- progressive muscular atrophy (PMA)
    - wasting
    - weakness
    - fasciculation
- progressive bulbar palsy
    - as PMA, but in distribution of motor cranial nerves
- pseudo-bulbar palsy
    - upper motor neurone disease affecting motor cranial nerve territory
- mixed type most common

Investigation
- EMG and muscle biopsy → denervation

Treatment
- no specific therapy
- supportive measures only
    - aspiration pneumonias common in bulbar and pseudo-bulbar palsy
- avoidance of contractures

Multiple Myeloma

Definition: a malignant proliferation of plasma cells
Incidence: about 4 per 100 000 per year

Clinical features
    anaemia
    bone pain
    pathological fracture
    hypercalcaemia
    peripheral neuropathy
    amyloidosis
    renal failure (related to tubular deposits of myeloma protein, amyloid or hypercalcaemia)
    hyperviscocity syndrome
    increased susceptibility to infection
    cord compression (from vertebral collapse or myeloma deposits)

Investigations
    ESR very high
    anaemia frequent
    monoclonal band on plasma protein electrophoresis,
    cf. other causes of monoclonal band
        localized plasmacytoma
        lymphoma
        Hodgkin's disease
        Waldenstrom's macroglobulinaemia
        benign monoclonal gammopathy
    Bence–Jones protein – 50%
    increased number of abnormal plasma cells in marrow
    osteolytic lesions in skeleton, especially skull

Treatment
    melphalan + prednisone: intermittent therapy
        $10\,mg/m^2/day$ melphalan
        $60\,mg/m^2/day$ prednisolone
        4 day courses, repeated initially at 6 week intervals
    hyperuricaemia prevented with allopurinol in association with chemotherapy
    local irradiation for bone pain
    anaemia – transfusion
    treat intercurrent infections
    hypercalcaemia – see p. 105
    plasmaphoresis may be employed in hyperviscocity syndrome

Monitor
    blood count with chemotherapy
    renal function
    immunoglobulin levels to assess efficacy of therapy
    serum calcium

Presentation of malignancy in the elderly can be
    asymptomatic
    masked by other illnesses
    with non-metastatic complications e.g.
        neuropathy
        depression
        dementia

Bronchogenic
    squamous cell, adenocarcinoma, anaplastic, bronchioalveolar
    major cancer of old age
    incidence approx. 250 per 100 000 per year
    mortality – accounts for approximately $1/6$ of all deaths at age 65
      and over
    aetiology
        smoking
        occupational exposure to
            radioactive gases
            asbestos
            arsenic
            nickel
            chromates
            metallic iron and iron oxides
            coal gas manufacture
    clinical features
        cough, dyspnoea, chest pain
        haemoptysis, weight loss, anorexia
        finger clubbing, hypertrophic osteoarthropathy
        pressure effects
            Horner's syndrome (sympathetic chain)
            hoarseness (recurrent laryngeal)
            superior vena caval syndrome
            Pancoast's tumour (brachial plexus)
            elevated diaphragm (phrenic nerve)
        thrombophlebitis migrans
        endocrine hormone secretion
            ACTH
            vasopressin
            parathyroid hormone
            TSH
            gonadotrophins

non-metastatic neurological presentations
        encephalitis
        myopathy
        cerebellar degeneration
        peripheral neuropathy
diagnosis made using
        chest X-rays
        sputum cytology
        tomography
        bronchoscopy
treatment
        usually symptomatic
        overall 5 year survival 5-7%

Breast carcinoma
    incidence – approx. 190 per 100 000 per year in females
    presentation
        breast lump ± secondaries
        Paget's disease of the breast
    treatment
        lumpectomy or simple mastectomy ± DXT
        radiotherapy for fungating mass
        metastatic spread
            oestrogens
            chemotherapy
            adrenalectomy
            or hypophysectomy ±
            analgesics

Oesophageal carcinoma
    almost always squamous cell
    incidence increases with age (approx. 30 per 100 000 per year)
    more common in men
    carcinoma in upper part common in patients with sideropenia

    carcinoma in middle part common in patients with achalasia

    other aetiological factors
        nitrosamines in food
        alcohol and tobacco
        tylosis
        chronic oesophagitis

presentation
    chest pain
    dysphagia
    aspiration pneumonia
treatment
    usually conservative
    radiotherapy or surgery occasionally used

Stomach (gastric carcinoma)
    incidence – third most common malignancy: 110 per 100000
        per year
    aetiology
        unknown but increased incidence in patients with chronic
            atrophic gastritis and PA
        genetic predisposition with blood group A
    presentation
        indigestion
        weight loss
        vomiting
        abdominal pain
        abdominal mass
        confusion
        anaemia
        haematemesis and melaena
        gastric ulcer responding poorly to medical treatment
    diagnosis confirmed by barium meal and endoscopy
    prognosis poor

    treatment – usually palliative

Carcinoma of rectum and colon: mortality 17000 per year in UK

Colonic carcinoma
    adenocarcinoma
    low grade malignancy
    incidence – approx 110 per 100000 per year
    aetiology
        low fibre diet
        polyp
        ulcerative colitis
    presentation
        symptoms vague
        change in bowel habit
        abdominal pain

weight loss
malaise
anaemia
symptoms of perforation – rarely
diagnosis made on
barium enema findings
colonoscopy
laparotomy
treatment
surgical resection
overall 5-year survival after resection is approx. 50%

Rectal carcinoma
adenocarcinoma
incidence: approx 75 per 100 000 per year
presentation
rectal bleeding
tenesmus
diarrhoea
faecal incontinence – may be the presenting complaint
diagnosis – protoscopy and biopsy
treatment
local excision if possible
abdominoperineal or anterior resection
local irradiation if mass large and involves deeper tissues
and patient is not fit for surgery

Prostatic carcinoma
most common malignancy of men over 65
incidence rises with age (approaching 100% as pre-invasive
carcinoma histologically in the higher age ranges)
reported incidence: 190 per 100 000 per year in men
presentation
asymptomatic – discovered on PR examination
retention of urine
renal failure
bone pain from metastases
acid phosphatase>0.7 U/l especially in those with local or distal
spread (NB not to be estimated within 24 hours of PR examination)
treatment
prostatectomy – TUR
oestrogens – used as an addition to surgery as well as by

itself to relieve (i) bone pain and (ii) to shrink carcinoma
and thus relieve ureteric obstruction caused by tumour
radiotherapy to tumour as well as metastases
orchidectomy – can be used instead of oestrogen
prognosis: 44% survive 5–years if no spread present at time of
diagnosis

Bladder carcinoma
incidence: approx. 70 per 100 000 per year
multifocal
papillary or solid
predisposing factors
stone
leukoplakia
aromatic amines
smoking
presentation
haematuria
abdominal pain

diagnosis confirmed by cystoscopy and biopsy
treatment
diathermy for papillomata
irradiation – supravoltage
local radioactive implant
cystectomy – partial or total with ileal conduit is the
treatment of choice but only rarely can it be performed in
the elderly

Kidney: hypernephroma
incidence: 5 per 100 000 per year
clinical features
asymptomatic or
haematuria
abdominal pain may be present in ½
abdominal mass
**pyrexia of unknown origin with leukocytosis common
confusion**
hypertension – only in rare renin-secreting tumours arising
from juxtaglomerular apparatus
polycythaemia
peripheral neuropathy
symptoms arising from metastatic spread

diagnosis
  plain X-rays of abdomen may show calcification
  IVP
  ultrasound – distinguishes simple cyst from solid tumour
  arteriogram – 'tumour blush'
treatment
  nephrectomy – in some even pulmonary metastases
    regress after nephrectomy
  for metastatic spread
    androgens
    vinblastine
prognosis – variable

Skin
Basal cell epithelioma
rodent ulcer
predisposing factors – actinic radiation; epidermal naevi;
  xeroderma pigmentosum
painless
commonly found on face, neck, auricle etc.
indurated margin
rarely metastasizes
treatment
  surgery
    curretage
    cryosurgery
  radiotherapy

Squamous cell carcinoma
arises in premalignant sundamaged skin (solar keratoses)
in situ tumour – Bowen's disease
malignant – metastasizes
(cf. keratoacanthoma
  benign
  rapidly growing
  dome shaped
  central keratinous plug
  resolves in approximately 8 months
  no therapy required)
treatment
  surgical excision
  radiotherapy if only single lesion
  for metastases: systemic chemotherapy and local per-
    fusion

Malignant melanoma
   arises from melanocytes
   sundamaged skin predisposes to development *de novo*
   arises in existing naevus

   metastasizes
   treatment
      local excision ± block dissection
      chemotherapy

Mycosis fungoides
   cutaneous lymphoma (usually reticulum cell sarcoma or lymphoblastic lymphoma, or Hodgkin's lymphoma)
   'T' lymphocytes
   in early stages resembles eczema or psoriasis
   later infiltrated plaques or ulcers develop
   in some erythroderma also develops
   diagnosis made by biopsy
   treatment
      topical application of dilute mechlorethamine
      irradiation
      systemic cytotoxic therapy

Leukaemias

Acute leukaemia
   usually myeloblastic
   may follow aplastic anaemia, paroxysmal nocturnal haemoglobinuria, myelofibrosis, chronic myeloid leukaemia, polycythaemia rubra vera
   clinical features
      fatigue
      anaemia
      weight loss, haemorrhage; tissue infiltration
   acute illness may be precipitated by infection
   prognosis poor
   treatment
      response to treatment not good but agents in combination have been tried e.g. daunorubicin, cystosine arabinoside and thioguanine

Chronic lymphatic
   incidence rises with age
   white cell count 50–100 × 10^9/litre
   asymptomatic

may present with
  anaemia
  lymphadenopathy
  splenomegaly ± hepatomegaly
  liability to recurrent infections
  haemolytic anaemia
  thrombocytopaenia
  monoclonal gammopathy
  herpes zoster
treatment
  chlorambucil ($0.1-0.2$ mg kg^{-1} day^{-1}) or cyclophospha-
    mide if symptoms present
  steroids for haemolytic anaemia and thrombocytopaenia +
  supportive measures e.g. blood transfusions, antibiotics
    for infection

Chronic myeloid
  malignant proliferation of granulocytes
  presentation
    anaemia
    weakness
    recurrent infections
    haemorrhagic tendency
    later lymphadenopathy
    splenomegaly (but may be absent or minimal)
  WCC > 100 000/mm but can be less (cf. leukamoid reaction)
  segmented neutrophils
  leukocyte alkaline phosphatase low, serum B$_{12}$ high
  platelets increased; later thrombocytopenia may develop
  bone marrow infiltrated by abnormal cells
  treatment
    busulphan – initial dose 4 mg/day (maintenance dose
      2 mg/day)
    hydroxyurea – dose 20 mg kg^{-1} day^{-1}
    irradiation of spleen if grossly enlarged
    supportive measures

Leukamoid reaction
  secondary
    to infection
      pneumococcal
      meningococcal
      tuberculosis
    malignancy especially with spread

leukocytes have normal or high alkaline phosphatase
bone marrow does not show abnormal cells
absence of philadelphia chromosome

Chronic myelomonocytic leukaemia
usually presents insidiously
but can present with acute illness
blood film – monocytosis with leukopenia and thrombocytopenia

bone marrow
hypercellular with large numbers of partly differentiated
cells;
sideroblasts may precede or accompany illness
prognosis better than CML (chronic myeloid)
5-year survival good even with supportive measures

Polycythaemia rubra vera
myeloproliferative disorder associated with inappropriate
proliferation of red cells
clinical features
red cell mass↑
WCC↑
leukocyte alkaline phosphatase↑
platelets↑
serum B₁₂↑
splenomegaly
hyperviscosity syndrome
haemorrhage – common complication
pruritus
treatment
venesection
^{32}P – dose depends on size of patient and degree of
polycythaemia
melphalan
of complications
iron for anaemia due to blood loss from gut
anticoagulants for vascular thrombosis
allopurinol for hyperuricaemia
cholestyramine for pruritus
(cf. secondary erythrocytosis
dehydration
stress
tissue anoxia, altitude

renal disease
cerebellar haemangioma
other tumours – renal, adrenal, hepatic
androgens etc.)

Primary myelofibrosis
fibrosis and new bone formation
extramedullary erythropoesis
leukoerythroblastic anaemia – immature red and white cells
found in blood
hepatosplenomegaly
trephine biopsy diagnostic – increased collagen and reticulum
fibres with reduced cellular content
may present with malignant phase
treatment
blood transfusion for anaemia
splenectomy if hypersplenism present
steroids, busulphan and androgens can be tried (give some
success)
(cf. secondary myelofibrosis
tuberculosis
metastases
chronic infection etc.)

Essential thrombocythaemia
malignant proliferation of platelets
platelet count↑
platelets abnormal in form and function
haemorrhage
thrombosis
splenomegaly
leukocyte alkaline phosphatase↑
serum B_{12}↑
bone marrow: increased number of abnormal megakaryocytes
treatment
^{32}P
busulphan
(NB splenectomy contraindicated)
(cf. secondary thrombocytosis
rheumatoid arthritis
carcinoma
Hodgkin's disease
haemorrhage
post-splenectomy
splenic vein thrombosis, etc.)

Normal Pressure Hydrocephalus

Aetiology
>
> not known but basic pathology is block in intracranial sub-arachnoid space due to diffuse fibrosis. Few are secondary to subarachnoid haemorrhage
>
> CSF pressure <180 mmHg

Clinical features
>
> **rapidly evolving signs and symptoms of dementia**
> **spastic ataxia (may cause repeated falls)**
> **incontinence of urine and faeces**
> diagnosis confirmed by
>
>> computerized transverse axial scanning which shows dilated ventricles with no dilatation of sulci; or
>>
>> air encephalogram, or
>>
>> $^{99}Tc^m$ – labelled albumin scinticisternography – at 24 hours cerebral ventricles are seen with no radioactivity over the surface.

Treatment
>
> symptomatic if NPH is secondary to subarachnoid haemorrhage as some recover spontaneously
>
> shunt
>
>> ventriculoatrial
>>
>> lumbar subarachnoid space to peritoneum or jugular vein or right atrium
>
> **NB not all improve with the shunt**

Osteomalacia

Definition: defective bone mineralization

Incidence: 4% of hospital admissions have osteomalacia

Aetiology
- vitamin D deficiency
  - malnutrition
  - lack of ultraviolet light
  - malabsorption
  - post-gastrectomy
- abnormal vitamin D metabolism
  - barbiturate therapy (liver enzyme induction)
  - liver disease
  - renal disease
- miscellaneous
  - malignant tumours
  - hypophosphataemia
- **in elderly the aetiology is multifactorial**

Clinical features
- bone pain
- bone tenderness
- muscle weakness – usually proximal but can be distal
- **general ill health**
- **fractures – osteomalacia responsible for 20–30% of fracture neck of femurs**
- serum calcium↓
- serum phosphate↓
- serum alkaline phosphatase↑

- vitamin D test – i.v. injection of D_3 produces a rise of $>25\%$ in fasting serum phosphate after five days in vitamin D deficient patients
- 25-hydroxycholecalciferol ↓
- X-rays
  - Looser's zones (pseudofractures) – diagnostic but only seen in minority
  - fractures
  - excessive intracortical resorption of phalanges due to secondary hyperparathyroidism
  - coarser trabecula in thin biconcave vertebrae

- isotopic scan
  - increased uptake generally by the skeleton
  - focal hot areas in the ribs

biopsy – excessive unmineralized osteoid tissue >40%

Treatment
    calcium with vitamin D tab BPC 1 t.d.s., or
    ultra-violet light
    in case of malabsorption large doses of vitamin D may be
       necessary. In these cases serum calcium level needs to be
       monitored regularly

Osteoporosis

Definition: reduction of bone tissue mass per volume

Aetiology
    primary – age +
        immobilization
        menopause (lack of oestrogens)
        ?lack of calcium
        ?lack of phosphate
    secondary
        Cushing's disease
        hyperparathyroidism
        hyperthyroidism
        diabetes mellitus
        excess steroid ingestion
        bone marrow involvement e.g.
            multiple myeloma
            carcinomatosis

Clinical features
    none (asymptomatic) to
    bone pain especially backache
    fractures (crush, neck of femur etc.)
    nerve root compression
    kyphosis
    loss of height
    loss of bone density on X-rays
    serum calcium, phosphate and alkaline phosphatase are usually
        normal
    biopsy: reduction in bone tissue mass per volume

Treatment
    for primary
        avoid immobilization +
        oestrogens – stilboestrol 1–3 mg daily (NB side effects in
            the elderly – oedema; withdrawal uterine bleeding etc.)

        anabolic steroids instead of oestrogens can be tried with
            some benefit – nandrolone decanoate 25 mg i.m. three
            injections at two week intervals

        oral calcium if calcium intake is low in the patient

        vitamin D with calcium and fluoride have also been tried
            with some success

    for secondary – treat the underlying cause

Paget's Disease

10% of elderly over 90 y have this on radiology

Aetiology – unknown

Clinical features
- none to
- bone pain (bones most commonly involved are sacrum, pelvis, tibiae, femora, spine and skull)
- bone deformity (skull enlargement, bowing of tibiae)
- high output failure
- blindness
- deafness
- osteogenic sarcoma

Investigations
- serum calcium and phosphate: normal
- serum alkaline phosphatase↑
- urinary hydroxyproline↑
- X-rays – lytic areas, zones of increased density, loss of trabecular pattern, deformity
- isotopic scan – increased uptake by areas involved by the disease (useful in monitoring progress with treatment)

Treatment
- given if there is extensive disease with pain, neurological complications or heart failure
- use calcitonin or mithramycin, or glucagon or diphosphonate
- calcitonin
    - inhibits excessive bone formation and relieves pain
    - 160 IU daily in divided doses i.m. or s.c.
    - response monitored by alkaline phosphatase level
- mithramycin
    - inhibits RNA synthesis
    - 25 mg kg^{-1} day^{-1} by i.v. infusion for 10 days; repeated 2–3 months later if disease remains
    - remission up to one year can be obtained
    - main toxic effects of the drug are on kidney, liver and platelets
- glucagon – 8–10 mg/day – after two weeks reduce to 2–3 mg subcutaneously once or twice a day
- diphosphonate – 7.5–20 mg kg^{-1} day^{-1}
- local irradiation especially in case of spinal involvement may be useful
- for pain indomethacin also has been found to be useful

Pancreatic Disease

Acute pancreatitis
    Aetiology
        idiopathic
        biliary tract disease
        hypercalcaemia
        hypothermia
        steroids
        mumps
    Clinical features
        asymptomatic to
        abdominal pain – lower abdominal with radiation to back
        nausea and vomiting
        confusion
        unconsciousness – a common presentation
        shock
        abdominal mass if pseudocyst present
        ↑serum amylase (cf. raised levels also found in
            perforation of ulcer
            dissecting aneurysm
            parotitis
            cholecystitis
            renal failure)
    Treatment
        fluid replacement
        analgesia for pain
        nasogastric tube for duodenal aspiration
        aprotinin may occasionally be useful – 500 000 KIU i.v.
            slowly followed by 200 000 KIU four hourly by infusion
        surgery if pseudocyst present

Chronic pancreatitis – end result of repeated attacks of acute pancreatitis
    Clinical features
        pain
        vomiting
        malabsorption
        jaundice
        hyperglycaemia (diabetes)
        X-rays may show calcification
        diagnosis can be made on ultrasound or ERCP findings

Treatment
    pancreatic extract if malabsorption present
    analgesia for pain
    occasionally pancreatectomy

Pancreatic carcinoma – accounts for about 3% of all tumours in old
age
    head: painless jaundice
    body or tail: bruit in abdomen due to obstruction of splenic vein
        may be audible
    tumours from both region may present with
        anorexia
        weight loss
        general ill health
        back pain
        deep vein thrombosis (repeated attacks)
        diagnosis made by hypotonic duodenogram in case of
            tumour of head of pancreas, although ultrasound and
            ERCP are investigations of choice
Treatment
    conservative unless tumour resectable
    in some palliative surgery i.e. bypass operation may be
        tried

Paraphrenia

Schizophrenia-like illness occuring in the elderly

Confined to women who are spinsters and emotionally remote

$1/5$ have family history of schizophrenia

Illness has two stages
    stage 1
        patient is irritable and suspicious and complains of tiredness, weakness and weight loss.

    stage 2
        auditory and visual hallucinations
        persecutory delusions – may accuse doctor or neighbour of sexual attack
        gross affect changes of young schizophrenics not seen in the elderly

Treatment – phenothiazines

Parkinson's Disease

Loss of pigmented neurones in substantia nigra

Common biochemical findings include dopamine deficiency and excess of cholinergic transmission.

Incidence: all types: 1–1.5 per 1000 of adult population

Aetiology
    idiopathic
    encephalitis
    manganese poisoning
    trauma
    progressive supranuclear palsy (Steele–Richardson syndrome – in addition to Parkinsonism these patients have upward gaze palsy, ataxia and dementia)
    drugs
        phenothiazines (block dopamine receptors)
        butyrophenones
        tetrabenazine
        reserpine
    carbon monoxide poisoning

Clinical features
    rigidity which may be cogwheel
    shuffling gait
    tremor
    bradykinesia
    expressionless face
    micrographia
    glabellar tap +ve
    excessive salivation
    dysphagia
    heartburn
    constipation
    complications
        immobility
        falls
        hypokinesia

Treatment
        levadopa with carbidopa (= sinemet) – use 110 mg sinemet tab. on alternate days; and increase by ½ tablet every 2–3 days until maximum benefit achieved

NB side effects of levadopa)
  nausea and vomiting
  confusion, psychoses
  hypotension
  dystonia
  'on-off' phenomenon
anticholinergics
  benzhexol 6–8 mg/day
  benapryzine 50 mg t.d.s. or q.d.s. – particularly effective
    against tremor
if levadopa not suitable amantadine or bromocriptine can be tried
for tremor stereotaxic surgery is useful
for severe hypokinesia in a stabolized parkinsonian patient try
  benztropine 2 mg or phenadrine 40 mg i.m.
for hyperpyrexia which can result from infection in patient on
  anticholinergics – i.v. mixture of pethidine, promethazine and
  chlorpromazine

Peptic Ulceration

Aetiology
     oesophageal ulcer – oesophageal reflux
     gastric ulcer
         ?reduction in protective mucus
         ?biliary reflux
         ?mucosal ischaemia
         ?gastric stasis
         (incidence 5.2–8.5%)

     duodenal ulcer – increased acid production in $1/3$

     specific causes of peptic ulceration
         hypercalcaemia from any cause
         Zollinger–Ellison syndrome
         renal dialysis – defective removal of gastrin

Clinical features
     asymptomatic
     anorexia
     weight loss
     vague abdominal pain
     dyspepsia
     nausea
     confusion especially associated with bleeding or perforation
     large gastric benign ulcer common in elderly

     complications
         more common and serious in the elderly (mortality high)
         bleeding
         perforation
             in elderly abdomen may not be rigid
             confusion may be the presentation
         stricture
             oesophageal stricture
             pyloric stenosis

         neoplasm especially in case of gastric ulcer

Treatment of ulcer
     antacids (aluminium hydroxide or magnesium trisilicate) for
         symptomatic relief
     cimetidine (H_2 receptor antagonist) 200 mg t.d.s. and 400 mg
         nocte – heals ulcer
     NB carbenoxolone likely to produce metabolic disturbance in
         elderly, therefore it should not be used)

Treatment of complications
 bleeding
  blood transfusion + cimetidine
  surgery if bleeding can not be controlled
 perforation
  surgery primarily
  conservative (drip, suck and antibiotics) in poor surgical
   risk patients
 pyloric stenosis – surgery
 peptic oesophageal stricture – dilatation or surgery

Peripheral Neuropathy

Definition: abnormal function of nerves due to disease of peripheral nerves (NB with age, nerve conduction velocity falls)

Aetiology
    mononeuropathy
        polyarteritis nodosa
        leprosy
    polyneuropathy
        metabolic
            diabetes mellitus
            amyloid
            dysproteinaemias
                myeloma
                cryoglobulinaemia
                Waldenström's macroglobulinaemia
            renal failure
            alcohol
        infections
            diphtheria
            tetanus
            Guillain-Barré
            infectious mononucleosis
        deficiency states – B_1, B_6, B_{12}, folic acid
        drugs
            nitrofurantoin
            isoniazid

        toxins
            heavy metals
            arsenic

        miscellaneous
            rheumatoid arthritis
            other connective tissue diseases
            sarcoidosis
            carcinoma – neuropathy tends to be of quick onset
            idiopathic – most commonly diagnosed
    entrapment neuropathy
        carpal tunnel syndrome (median nerve)
        ulnar nerve compression
        radial nerve – 'saturday night palsy'
        meralgia paresthesia (lateral femoral cutaneous nerve)
        Morton's metatarsalgia (caused by pressure on planter nerves)

Clinical features of polyneuropathy
    numbness or pain in hands and feet
    may also complain of burning feet
    unsteadiness
    sensory objective signs may be equivocal in the elderly
    reflexes diminished or absent

Treatment
    treat the underlying cause if possible
    in large number no cause may be found for the neuropathy –
        try empirically a course of steroids in these cases

Peripheral Vascular Disease

Aetiology
    atheroma
    embolus
    diabetic microangiopathy
    giant cell arteritis
    vasculitis with connective tissue disorders
    Buerger's disease
    cold injury
    β-blocking drugs
    dysproteinaemias and other states increasing blood viscosity
        may precipitate symptoms

Clinical features
    asymptomatic
    intermittent claudication
    cold feet
    parasthaesiae in feet
    rest pain
    large vessel bruits
    localized aneurysm formation
    loss of peripheral pulses
    cyanosis
    gangrene
    ischaemic ulcers
    NB exclude 'intermittent claudication of cauda equina'

Treatment
    stop β-blocking drugs
    asymptomatic – advise foot care
    ischaemia of limb – anticoagulants and/or vascular surgery
    ulcer with cellulitis – antibiotics
    dry gangrene – allow autoamputation
    gangrene; extensive/wet/gas – amputation
    rehabilitation post-surgery with rapid fitting of limb if necessary
        when stump satisfactory
    high proportion of elderly amputees fail to walk
    home assessment and early adaptation is necessary

Peripheral Vascular Disease of Upper Limb

Aetiology
    sclerodema
    arteritis with connective tissue disease
    axillary artery compression, cervical rib etc
    giant cell arteritis
    embolus
    very rarely atheroma
    dissecting aneurysm of aortic arch

Pneumonia

Incidence: high, often a terminal illness in the elderly

Aetiology
    viral – influenza, cytomegalovirus, measles etc.
        NB – often pneumonia is due to secondary bacterial infection
    bacterial
        Streptococcus pneumoniae—commonest organism
        Haemophilus influenzae
        Staphylococcus aureus
        Klebsiella pneumonia · Friedlander's pneumonia
        Pseudomonas aeruginosa
        Proteus
        E. coli
        Mycobacterium tuberculosis – see p. 164 etc.
        Mycoplasma pneumoniae – see p. 56
        Chlamydia psittaci – psittacosis
        Coxiella burneti – Q fever
    fungi – *Actinomyces israeli* etc.
    (cf. lipoid pneumonia)
        reaction to mineral oil (paraffin oil)
        diagnosis made on X-rays and on staining of sputum with
            sudan dye
    aspiration pneumonia
        reaction to gastric contents
        'Mendelson's syndrome'
        treatment – O_2, hydrocortisone and ampicillin

Clinical features
    tachypnoea
    tachycardia
    confusion
    fever may be absent in early stages
    sputum may be absent or scanty
    chest signs may be absent or minimal
    X-rays – mottled shadowing rather than homogeneous seen in
        younger patients
    organism can be isolated by blood culture

    complications
        lung abscess
        empyema
        congestive heart failure
        cardiac arrhythmias
        pericarditis
        shock etc.

Treatment
antibiotic
start with ampicillin 0.5–1 g q.d.s.
change according to sensitivities of organism isolated
and/or patient's response

**physiotherapy – very important in those who can not cough
up sputum by themselves**
treat arrhythmias or heart failure if present
if shock present – steroids

Polymyalgia Rheumatica

A collagen disease

Clinical features
- shoulder pain with tenderness
- difficulty in combing hair
- nocturnal and early morning exacerbations
- pyrexia – low grade
- anorexia
- malaise
- ESR >40 mm/h but often >100 mm/h
- normochromic normocytic anaemia
- raised serum immunoglobulins
- **associated with temporal arteritis** – temporal artery changes found in 20–50% of patients; arteries are tender and thickened with loss of pulsation

Treatment
- **steroids**
  - start with prednisolone 40–60 mg/day
  - reduce at weekly intervals by 2.5–5 mg until ESR <30 mm/h
- treatment usually given for about 18 months – longer if the condition relapses

Definition: fall of systolic BP > 20 mmHg with symptoms (About 11% of elderly have postural BP fall>20 mmHg)

Aetiology
  - **idiopathic (autonomic failure)**
  - **Parkinsonism**
  - **Shy-Drager syndrome (autonomic degeneration with Parkinsonism)**
  - **cerebrovascular disease**
  - **polyneuropathy – associated with**
    - diabetes mellitus
    - B_{12} deficiency
    - carcinoma
    - alcoholism
    - tabes dorsalis
    - Guillain–Barré syndrome
  - cerebral tumour
  - **drugs**
    - hypotensive agents (especially post-ganglionic sympathetic blockers)
    - tricyclic antidepressants
    - barbiturates
    - anticholinergic agents
    - phenothiazines
    - levadopa
    - bromocriptine
    - diuretics
    - vasodilators
    - a-blocking agents

Clinical features
  - **on standing**
    - **dizziness**
    - **weakness**
    - **clouding of consciousness**
    - **confusion**
    - **falls**
  - NB exercise – induced hypotension similar presentation

Treatment
  - **withdraw possible precipitating drugs**
  - elastic stockings
  - slow sodium tablets ⎤
  - 9-a-fludrocortisone ⎦ NB excessive fluid retention hazard
  - dihydroergotamine – vasoconstrictor

Pressure Sores (Decubitus Ulcers)

Classification

Superficial: good prognosis if actively treated to prevent progression
Deep: tissue loss inevitable.

or

Temperature difference between affected area and surrounding skin <1°C, >2.5°C

Predisposing factors

compression and shearing forces in combination with:
poor tissue perfusion
immobility and paresis
general poor health
poor nutrition
anaemia
hypoxaemia
incontinence - skin maceration

Treatment/prevention

frequent turning of immobile patients
ripple (alternating pressure) bed
water bed
net bed
'low loss' air bed
sheepskin pads
bed cradles for feet
catheterization if prolonged contact with urine results from incontinence

Local

dressing after Eusol, cetrimide or other antiseptic agents
oxygen
ultraviolet light
surgical debridement
dextranomer powder (Debrisan)
streptokinase/streptodornase - useful when necrotic tissue present

General

improve nutrition
correct anaemia, heart failure, oedema etc.
ascorbic acid 200–500 mg daily
oral zinc sulphate 220 mg t.d.s.

Pulmonary Embolism

Accounts for 3-4% of all hospital admissions
Mortality 10-20%

Aetiology
>   deep vein thrombosis (**often not clinically evident**)

Clinical features
>   acute
>>   dyspnoea of sudden onset
>>   tachycardia
>>   cardiac dysrhythmia; especially atrial fibrillation
>>   hypotension
>>   pleuritic pain or
>>   haemoptysis if pulmonary infarction occurs
>>   heart failure
>>   syncope
>   chronic
>>   progressive dyspnoea
>>   cor pulmonale

Investigations
>   chest X-ray: nil change to
>>   collapse
>>   consolidation
>>   effusion
>>   regional oligaemia
>>   cardiomegaly
>   ECG
>>   nil change to S_1 Q_3 T_3 (S wave in lead I, q wave in lead III with T wave inversion in lead III)
>>   right ventricular strain pattern

>   isotopic lung scan: perfusion and ventilation
>>   normal or
>>   regional under-perfusion, but normal aeration – positive in 77-84%

Treatment
>   anticoagulants
>>   heparin by i.v. infusion – controlled by calcium thrombin time, followed by warfarin orally – controlled by pro-thrombin time
>>   alternatively streptokinase or urokinase

NB hazards of anticoagulants in the presence of
    hypertension
    cerebrovascular disease
    active gastro-intestinal disease
modify dose of warfarin in the presence of
    hepatic disease
    congestive cardiac failure
    concomitant drug therapy known to alter effectiveness of
        coumarin anticoagulants

Pulmonary Tuberculosis

Incidence – high: 1.8% (active TB) at autopsy

Aetiology – *Mycobacterium tuberculosis*

Clinical features
  common in males
  usually a reactivation of old TB focus
  symptoms
    non-specific and slow progressing
    general malaise
    weight loss
    mild temperature (PUO) etc.
  chest X-rays
    can be normal – 'cryptic miliary TB' (particularly common in elderly)
    upper lobe shadowing
    miliary shadowing
  diagnosis made on
    clinical signs and symptoms
    radiology
    skin testing (NB. **skin test can be negative in early stages, in chronically ill elderly and in acute miliary TB**)
    sputum – staining and microscopy, culture
    culture of biopsy material from:
        bone marrow
        liver
        lymph node

Treatment
  isoniazid 300 mg/day +
  rifampicin 450 mg/day +
  ethambutol 15 mg kg^{-1} day^{-1} for first two months
  (NB
      treatment should be given for at least nine months
      side effects of therapy
          isoniazid
              peripheral neuropathy
              hepatitis
          ethambutol
              retrobulbar neuritis
          rifampicin
              allergic thrombocytopenic purpura
              cholestatic jaundice)

Pyrexia of Unknown Origin

Infections
   pneumonia
   urinary tract infection
   abscess
   endocarditis
   tuberculosis

Neoplasm
   lymphomas
   carcinomas (especially renal, hepatobiliary)

Connective tissue disorders
   giant cell arteritis
   polyarteritis nodosa
   systemic lupus erythematosus etc.

Miscellaneous
   pulmonary infarction
   myocardial infarction
   anaemia
   exposure to hot environment (especially if temperature
      regulatory mechanisms impaired – see heat stroke, p. 112)
   factitious fever

Investigations
   FBC
   ESR
   MSU
   liver function tests
   plasma protein electrophoresis
   immune complexes in serum
   chest X-ray
   blood cultures
   ECG
   suspected tuberculosis
      tuberculin test (useful if negative)
      early morning urine specimens for culture and microscopy
      sputum specimens for culture and microscopy
      see also p. 164
   if SLE suspected
      LE cell preparations
      antinuclear factor titre
      anti-DNA antibody titre

in addition
> biopsy of lymph node if enlarged
> intravenous pyelogram
> temporal artery biopsy if ESR raised
> liver biopsy and marrow aspiration for histology and culture if disseminated tuberculosis suspected

Renal Failure

Renal function falls with age
Normal blood urea 3.9–9.9 mmol/l
Normal creatinine 52–169 mmol/l

Aetiology

Acute

> dehydration
>> vomiting, diarrhoea, etc.
>
> hypotension
>> blood loss
>> myocardial infarction
>> pulmonary embolism
>> Gram-negative septicaemia etc.
>
> obstruction
>> urethral stricture
>> urethral carcinoma
>> prostate hypertrophy
>> prostate carcinoma
>> stone

drugs
> some sulphonamides
> cephaloridine
> amphotericin B
> tetracyclines
> aminoglycosides
> phenindione etc.

miscellaneous
> hypercalcaemia
> renal vein thrombosis – tumour, polycythaemia, amyloid
>> etc.
>
> renal artery thrombosis
> **acute necrotizing papillitis (not uncommon in elderly)**
>> associated with diabetes and vascular disease
>
> features:
>> haematuria, oliguria, fever, confusion, anaemia
>> papillae may be sloughed – ureteric colic

Chronic

> pyelonephritis – **chronic pyelonephritis said to be commonest
> renal disease in elderly, but pathological changes probably
> multi-factorial**

hypertension
diabetes mellitus
urate nephropathy
amyloid
prolonged hypercalcaemia (any cause see p. 00)
myeloma
analgesic nephropathy – papillary necrosis
chronic potassium depletion
chronic obstructive uropathy
glomerulonephritis (not common) – acute glomerulonephritis
    may present with
      oedema
      congestive cardiac failure
      anorexia
      nausea
      vomiting
      diarrhoea
      haematuria
      proteinuria
      microscopy of urine: red cell casts
      renal biopsy necessary for diagnosis

Treatment
Acute
    rehydrate
    maintain fluid input equal to output + 500 ml until recovery
    treat infection if present
    treat underlying cause if possible
    treat hyperkalaemia if present
    dialysis in selected cases with potentially reversible cause of
      acute renal failure

Chronic
    treat infection if present
    correct obstruction if present
    withdraw analgesics associated with nephropathy if analgesic
      nephropathy diagnosed
    aim to keep patient as free of symptoms as possible (low
      protein diet if symptoms diminished by this means)
      antiemetics
      aluminium hydroxide to lower phosphate
      intermittent blood transfusion for symptomatic anaemia
      (NB transfusion raises blood viscosity and thus dim-
        inishes renal perfusion – renal function may
        deteriorate)

Respiratory Failure

$PaO_2 < 2.8\,kPa$ $PaCO_2 > 6.3\,kPa$

(1) Hypoxaemia with CO_2 retention
   aetiology
      chronic bronchitis
      myasthenia gravis
      hypothermia
      Pickwickian syndrome
      polyneuropathy
      opiate intoxication
      barbiturate intoxication
   clinical features
      confusion
      drowsiness
      central cyanosis
      flapping tremor
      cardiac failure may be present
      fundal venous engorgement
      occasionally papilloedema
      wide pulse pressure

(2) Hypoxaemia without CO_2 retention
   aetiology
      chronic bronchitis (some cases)
      asthma (acute)
      pulmonary embolism
      pneumothorax
      pneumonia
      pulmonary oedema
      fibrosing alveolitis
      kyphoscolioscis

   clinical features
      confusion
      drowsiness
      central cyanosis
      cardiac failure may be present

   initial investigations
      chest X-ray and blood gases essential
      sputum for culture and sensitivity
      blood culture if infection suspected and there is no sputum

Management
  oxygen
      high concentration in hypoxaemia without CO_2 retention
      low concentration – in cases with CO_2 retention (24% oxygen initially, increasing if CO_2 retention not exacerbated – blood gases essential to monitor response)
  antibiotics if respiratory infection associated
  physiotherapy
  bronchial suction if excess secretions present
  bronchodilators for reversible airway obstruction
      preferably by aerosol inhalation
      parenteral or enteral administration otherwise ·
  diuretics for heart failure
  respiratory stimulants as temporary measure to aid physiotherapy
  steroids for reversible airways obstruction in severely ill patient or if bronchodilators are ineffective
  naloxone for opiate intoxication
  assisted ventilation if reversible disease present, particularly asthma or drug intoxication

Scurvy

Vitamin C deficiency

Clinical features
> **uncommon although deficiency common**
> sheet haemorrhages
> follicular hyperkeratosis with haemorrhages
> arthralgia (occasional joint effusions)
> fatigue
> megaloblastic anaemia
> swollen gums if own teeth present + gingival haemorrhages
> very rarely haemorrhage may occur in suborbital or subdural spaces
>
> leukocyte and serum ascorbic acid↓

Treatment
> ascorbic acid 0.5–1 g b.d. or t.d.s. for one week and then ascorbic acid tab BP (25 mg) one three times a day

Shoulder-Hand Syndrome

Painful stiff shoulder with tender swollen fingers and hand
    associated with
        myocardial infarction
        CVA
        trauma
        cervical disc lesion
    X-rays – patchy osteoporosis of head of humerus and wrist bones
    may lead to atrophy of muscles and contractures
    treatment – passive and active exercises

    cf. **adhesive capsulitis, supraspinatus tendinitis**

Adhesive capsulitis
    may follow
        myocardial infarction
        hemiplegia
        or pneumonia
    pain and tenderness in area of deltoid muscle
    inability to raise arm passively and actively
    X-rays
        normal in majority
        in long-standing cases – sclerosis of greater tuberosity may
          be seen

    may remit within 6–24 months
    treatment
        local heater cold therapy
        active exercises
        or intra-articular injection of hydrocortisone

Supraspinatus tendinitis
    follows an injury
    abduction painful – but full range of passive movements possible
    localized tenderness over supraspinatus tendon

    X-rays may show calcific deposits in the muscle

    treatment
        injection of hydrocortisone +
        physiotherapy

Small Bowel Diverticular Disease

(1) **Duodenal**
    incidence
        10–20% over 75
        site: mainly in second part of duodenum on concave border
        many embedded in pancreas
    aetiology
        unknown
        age related
    symptoms
        nil: occasionally dyspepsia
    complications
        haemorrhage (rare)
        perforation (rare)
        malabsorption (small bowel contamination)
        iron deficiency anaemia
    treatment
        rarely surgical if symptomatic (other pathology usually responsible)
        replacement of deficiencies

(2) **Jejunum**
    may be asymptomatic
    cause malabsorption and steatorrhoea by small bowel contamination

Stroke

Definition: an acute fall of cerebral function of presumed vascular origin with disability lasting>24 hours. If disability recovers within 24 hours then it is described as transient ischaemic attack (TIA).

Prevalence: 2 per 1000 population
Accounts for 10-20% of total mortality

Aetiology of TIA's
    atheroma
    emboli
        cardiac (infarction, arrhythmias, myxoma etc.)
        tumour
        fat
        dysproteinaemias
    hypotension
        myocardial infarction
        dysrhythmias
        postural hypotension
        pulmonary embolism
    miscellaneous
        anaemia
        polycythaemia (primary or secondary)
        thrombocythaemia
        respiratory failure
        systemic lupus erythematosis
        giant cell arteritis
        post-irradiation vasculopathy

Aetiology of completed stroke
    any of above causes +
    bleeding due to
        thrombocytopaenia
        anticoagulant therapy
        defibrination syndrome
            malignancy
            sepsis
            keto-acidosis
            incompatible transfusion
    subarachnoid haemorrhage
    (cf. subdural haematoma – p. 177
    intracranial tumours – p. 122

Clinical features
    vary according to blood vessel territory involved
    TIA's may present with
        weakness
        paraesthesiae
        blindness (amaurosis fugax)
        dysphasia
        hemianopia
        vertigo
        dysarthria
        drop attacks
        confusion etc.
    completed stroke
        symptoms depend on extent and site of brain damage
        may present with
            hemiparesis
            disturbance in cranial nerve territories
            sensory disturbance
            dysphasia
            confusion
            coma
            epilepsy
            death
        complications
            intellectual failure
            **incontinence - spontaneous continence may occur
                in 4-6 weeks**
            dysphagia
            spasticity
            contractures - if patient is not mobilized early
            pressure sores
            epilepsy
            depression
            persistent pain in arm and leg
            hypothermia

Treatment
    good nursing care
    **physiotherapy + occupational therapy ± speech therapy -
        most important - should be started as soon as possible to
        get maximum benefit as well as to prevent contractures**
    aspirin or anticoagulants for TIA's

surgery

> to restore patency of extracranial carotid arteries – those who might benefit must have a plaque with a narrowing of at least 70%
>
> to evacuate a localized clot

agents to reduce cerebral oedema are of little benefit in acute stroke

naftidofuryl may be of benefit

post-discharge care – patients with stroke are very liable to become depressed or frustrated once discharged home. They may require day centre attendance for mental stimulation or day hospital attendance if they are not physically independent enough to manage at home

Subdural Haematoma (chronic)

Collection of blood between dura and arachnoid spaces

Aetiology
> **trauma**
>> **may be trivial in the elderly**
>> **history may not be obtained since there is a long interval between trauma and symptoms**
>
> spontaneous

Clinical features
> **fluctuating consciousness** – slowness in thinking, confusion or drowsiness intermittent with normal mental state ±
> lateralizing signs
> ptosis and dilated pupil on affected side
> **may also present with stroke** (contralateral or ipsilateral), or **dementia**
> skull X-rays may show
>> displaced pineal
>> displaced choroid plexus
>> occasional fracture
>
> computer assisted tomography – positively localizes the haematoma
> CSF may be clear, xanthochromic or blood stained if recent contusion present

Treatment
> **evacuation through burr holes – this may be necessary before investigations can be performed if condition of the patient deteriorates rapidly and diagnosis is suspected clinically**

Tardive Dyskinesia

Definition
>   involuntary movement of tongue, mouth and facial muscles
>   ± choreiform movement of limbs
>   ± respiratory grunting

Prevalence: – said to lie between 0.5–50%

Aetiology
>   adverse reaction to drugs
>>   phenothiazines
>>   butyrophones
>>   metoclopramide
>>   tricyclic antidepressants etc.
>>   (NB dyskinesia reaction related to dose, time and age)
>   senile chorea

Treatment
>   stop the offending drug
>   short trial with one of the following may help
>>   tetrabenazine
>>   choline
>>   benzodiazepines
>>   baclofen

Prevention
>   avoid prolonged administration of drugs that are known to produce this
>   avoid usage of anticholinergics with neuroleptics

Thyrotoxicosis

Results from increased secretion of hormones T_4 and/or T_3
Incidence: accounts for 2-3% of hospital admissions

Aetiology
- diffuse goitre
- toxic nodular goitre
- toxic adenoma
- transient thyrotoxicosis associated with thyroiditis
- ectopic hormone production by tumour (bronchogenic) – rare

Clinical features
- **classical symptoms may be absent**
- **muscle weakness with cramps**
- **confusion**
- **depression (apathetic thyrotoxicosis)**
- weight loss
- **atrial fibrillation**
    - **$1/3$ of patients have AF**
    - **responds poorly to digoxin**
- congestive heart failure
- diarrhoea
- usually no goitre
- **ophthalmoplegia is rare in the elderly and only mild variety seen**
- occasionally patient may present with osteoporosis

Investigations
- $T_4 \uparrow$
- T_3 normal or high (in T_3 toxicosis only T_3 is raised) (T_3 rises later and less consistently in elderly)
- TRH test
    - useful in borderline cases
    - absent or flat response supports diagnosis

Treatment
- carbimazole
    - 10 mg eight hourly; reduce after 4–6 weeks to maintenance dose
    - treatment usually given for 18–24 months
- **radioactive iodine**
    - **^{131}I or ^{125}I treatment of choice for elderly who are going to be a problem with regard to taking tablets**
    - **NB risk of hypothyroidism post-treatment is high but risk is lower if ^{125}I is used than if ^{131}I**

surgery
    rarely used
    indicated if pressure effects present
beta-adrenergic blockers – used for symptomatic relief while
    waiting for laboratory results to confirm clinical diagnosis

Trigeminal Neuralgia (tic douloureux)

Recurrent paroxysms of pain in one or more territories of fifth cranial nerve
More common in females
Severity and frequency of pain may lead to suicide

Trigger factors
- touch
- chewing
- cold wind
- swallowing
- washing/shaving
- weight loss may occur through inability to eat

Treatment
- carbamazepine 100 mg daily initially, increasing gradually
- phenytoin 50–200 mg per day
  - these agents may suppress or shorten attacks
  - side-effects
    - carbamazepine – mainly drowsiness
    - phenytoin – mainly drowsiness, nystagmus, ataxia
- alcohol injection of Gasserian ganglion – relief in some cases for 1–2 years
- section of sensory part of V cranial nerve
- NB sensory loss over one side of face

Urinary Tract Infection

Commonest infection in the elderly
Usually only bladder or urethra involved

Incidence
    females > males
    over 65
        females at home 23%
        males at home 10%
        females in continuing care 34%
        males in continuing care 34%

Aetiology
    E. coli, Proteus, Pseudomonas, Klebsiella
    Streptococcus faecalis
    Staphylococcus etc.

Predisposing factors
    large residual urine
    cystocoele
    prostatic hypertrophy, prostatic carcinoma, urethral stricture
        etc.
    urethral obstruction from any cause
    catheterization
    atonic bladder
    diabetes mellitus
    bladder diverticula
    bladder stone
    vesico-colic fistula

Diagnosis
    colony count $>10^5$/ml
    >20 pus cells/ml

Clinical features
    asymptomatic
    nocturia
    frequency
    incontinence
    confusion
    dysuria (uncommon in elderly)
    renal failure
    septicaemia
    rigors (uncommon in elderly)

Treatment
    antibiotic – according to sensitivity
    in catheterized patient, eradication of infection unlikely –
    bladder irrigation with antiseptic solution preferable

Valvular Heart Disease

Aortic stenosis
    aetiology
        fibrous thickening
        calcific valves
        bicuspid aortic valve
        rheumatic heart disease

    clinical features
        asymptomatic
        dyspnoea on exertion
        angina
        syncope
        congestive heart failure
        narrow pulse pressure
        ejection murmur conducted to neck (**cf. aortic sclerosis mid-systolic murmur**)
    left ventricular hypertrophy

    treatment
        treat heart failure
        mild stenosis – no treatment
        severe – valve replacement
        if syncope occurs – indicates very severe disease – valve replacement indicated

Aortic incompetence
    aetiology
        rheumatic heart disease
        calcific valves
        giant cell arteritis
        bacterial endocarditis
        syphilitic aortitis
        dissecting aneurysm of aorta
        Marfan's disease and related disorders of connective tissue

    clinical features
        congestive heart failure
        collapsing pulse
        Corrigan's sign +ve
        early diastolic murmur at left sternal edge
        left ventricular enlargement
        occasionally Austin–Flint murmur (mid-diastolic murmur due to regurgitant flow impinging on mitral valve)

treatment
    treat failure
    if incompetence severe – valve replacement

Mitral stenosis (rare in elderly)
    aetiology
        rheumatic

    clinical features
        dyspnoea
        haemoptysis
        oedema
        chest pain
        atrial fibrillation
        systemic emboli – most commonly cerebral
        pulse diminished
        loud first sound
        may have opening snap
        mid-diastolic murmur
        left atrial enlargement

    investigations
        chest X-ray – may show calcified valve and enlarged left atrium
        right oblique chest X-ray with barium swallow confirms left atrial enlargement
        ECG – p mitrale, may show atrial fibrillation

    treatment
        diuretics for failure
        digoxin for atrial fibrillation .
        anticoagulants for prevention of systemic emboli
        valvotomy for severe stenosis leading to pulmonary hypertension
        valve replacement if valvotomy inappropriate

Mitral incompetence
    Aetiology
        papillary muscle dysfunction or infarction
        mitral valve prolapse
        chordae rupture
        rheumatoid arthritis
        Marfan's syndrome
        rheumatic heart disease etc.

clinical features
    tiredness
    chest pain
    palpitations
    heart failure
    pansystolic murmur at apex with radiation to axilla (may
        have mid-diastolic flow murmur)

treatment
    digoxin for rapid atrial fibrillation
    diuretics for heart failure
    for acute incompetence when medical treatment fails or for
        other selected cases, valve replacement may be ap-
        propriate

Viral Infections

Common cold
    upper respiratory tract infection
    may present with confusion
    may lead to severe bacterial infection

Influenza (A, B or C)
    upper respiratory tract infection
    clinical features
        cough, sneezing
        pyrexia
        muscle aches
        confusion
        prostration
        anorexia, nausea and constipation are frequently present
        may lead to
            serious bacterial infection
            hypotension
            myocarditis
            meningoencephalitis
            cranial nerve palsies
            hemiplegia
    treatment
        symptomatic
        antibiotic if bacterial infection develops

Herpes simplex
    cold sore
    tense vesicles with clear fluid
    5% IDU (idoxuridine) quickens resolution

Herpes zoster
    varicella causing virus
    disease of nerves of skin
        vesicles along dermatomes
        affects thoracic nerves in 55%
    fever and pain may appear 4–5 days before vesicles
    trigger factors
        malignancy
        radiotherapy
        cytotoxic drugs
        pressure on nerve roots

complications
- **post-herpetic neuralgia**
  - **common and severe in elderly**
  - **may lead to suicide**
  - **in 75% of elderly it is present for two months**
- secondary bacterial infection
- generalized zoster
- encephalomyelitis
- Bell's palsy if geniculate ganglion involved – Ramsey–Hunt syndrome

treatment
- **40% IDU may help post-herpetic neuralgia if treatment is started early**
- analgesics for pain
- antibiotics for secondary infection
- NB ophthalmic opinion if ophthalmic division of V involved

Viral hepatitis
- hepatitis A
  - common in community
  - may present with
    - confusion
    - anorexia
    - vomiting
    - abdominal pain
    - weight loss
    - jaundice – obstructive initially
    - hepatomegaly
    - splenomegaly in $1/3$
    - pruritus
- hepatitis B
  - has more insidious onset
  - high mortality
  - HBAg positive
- treatment
  - no specific treatment

Warts

Usually asymptomatic
Treatment
    liquid nitrogen for finger warts
    podophyllin for perianal warts

Investigations

Only those investigations that are going to affect the management of the patient should be performed.

General Screen for In-patients

full blood count
ESR
protein and strip
urine testing
urea and electrolytes
chest X-rays

NB
   ESR
      up to 40 mm/hour may be found in apparently healthy
         elderly
      normal low ESR may be present in association with disease
         e.g. malignancy, myocardial infarction etc.

Neutrophilia
      infections (pneumonia, UTI, cellulitis etc.)
      haemorrhage
      myocardial infarction
      haemolytic anaemia
      carcinoma
      gout
      diabetic ketoacidosis
      uraemia

Neutropenia
      with age there is tendency for WCC to fall
      normal range for the elderly – 3.0–8.5 × 10^9/1
      influenza
      overwhelming infection of any type
      hypoplastic anaemia
      hypersplenism (e.g. Felty's syndrome)
      typhoid fever
      vitamin B_{12} deficiency
      drugs
            alkylating agents
            colchicine ·
            phenylbutazone
            antithyroid drugs
            antihistamines
            gold salts

Eosinophilia
  parasitic infestation e.g. trichinosis
  polyarteritis nodosa
  asthma
  Hodgkin's disease, chronic myelocytic leukaemia
  polycythaemia rubra versa
  occasionally found in cases of carcinoma

Lymphocytosis
  viral infections
  brucellosis, tuberculosis
  leukaemias (lymphocytes abnormal)

Thrombocytopaenia
  idiopathic
  drug-induced – quinine, thiazides, gold etc.
  leukaemias
  carcinoma
  systemic lupus erythematosus (SLE)
  bacterial endocarditis
  diffuse i.v. coagulation
  uraemia, B_{12} deficiency
  hypersplenism

Urea and creatinine
  vary with age and weight
  low values may be found in patients with low protein intake,
    inappropriate ADH secretion etc.

Bicarbonate
  low (acidosis)
      uraemia
      ketoacidosis
      lactic acidosis
          diabetes mellitus
          septicaemia
      hypothermia
      drug induced – acetazolamide etc.
      (respiratory alkalosis)
  high (alkalosis)
      alkali therapy
      diuretic therapy
      respiratory acidosis
      potassium depletion

            Conn's syndrome
            Cushing's disease

Sodium
    low (hyponatraemia) see p. 111
    high (hypernatraemia)
            inadequate fluid intake
            excess fluid loss through skin – burns
            excess fluid loss from gut – diarrhoea
            excess saline administration
            hyperaldosteronism
            Cushing's syndrome

Potassium
    low see p. 110
    high (hyperkalaemia)
            renal failure
            administration of K-sparing diuretics
            Addison's disease
            diabetic ketoacidosis – in early stages

Albumin
    low
            general ill-health – (level reflects severity)
            liver disease
            renal disease
            malabsorption
            pressure sores
            burns
            inappropriate ADH secretion

Globulins
    there is general increase with age
    diffuse increase
            acute or chronic infection
            neoplasia
            autoimmune disease
            liver disease
    monoclonal band – see p. 129

Urinary
    proteinuria
            infection
            glomerulosclerosis
            diabetic nephropathy

analgesic nephropathy
myeloma
congestive heart failure
glomerulonephritis (rare)

haematuria
infection
trauma (catheter)
papilloma
renal carcinoma
subacute bacterial endocarditis
stone etc.

bilirubinuria
obstructive jaundice
hepatocellular disease

urobilinogen in urine
haemolysis
hepatocellular jaundice
pulmonary embolism
constipation
some cases of pernicious anaemia
large haematoma

Bone biochemistry
indicated in
malignant bone disease
suspected osteomalacia
suspected Paget's disease
renal failure
suspected hyperparathyroidism

NB
calcium falls with age in men
calcium rises with age in women

hypocalcaemia see p. 109
hypercalcaemia see p. 105
low phosphate
osteomalacia
hyperparathyroidism

high phosphate
renal failure
hypoparathyroidism
acromegaly

          vitamin D excess
          diabetic ketosis
high alkaline phosphatase
          osteomalacia
          Paget's disease
          fracture
          malignant bone disease
          chronic leg ulcers
          immobilization
          liver disease
          steatorrhoea
          giant cell arteritis
          senile cardiac amyloidosis

Liver function tests
    indicated in
        suspected liver disease
        jaundice
        hepatomegaly
        confusion
        coma
  NB
    bilirubin ↑
        liver disease
            hepatitis
            cirrhosis
            malignant disease – primary or secondary
            drugs see p. 00
        biliary obstruction
            stone ± infection
            tumour
                of bile duct
                of head of pancreas
            glands in porta hepatus

        pulmonary embolism
        haemolysis
        congestive heart failure
  SGOT↑
        haemolysis
        hepatocellular disease
        myocardial infarction
        occasionally in stroke and pulmonary embolism
        primary muscle disease

Hydroxybutyrate dehydrogenase (HBD)↑
    myocardial infarction (main indication) but may also be high in liver disease, muscle disease, megaloblastic anaemia, pulmonary embolism and stroke

Creatine phosphokinase (CPK)
    muscle disease (main indication)
    also raised in
        trauma (injection)
        pulmonary embolism
        pulmonary oedema
        CVA
        hypothyroidism

Thyroid function tests
    Hypothyroidism – T_4↓
        if result equivocal and diagnosis suspected clinically to do TSH (in primary hypothyroidism TSH is raised)
    Hyperthyroidism – T_4↑
        if result equivocal and diagnosis suspected clinically to do T_3
        if T_3 also equivocal to do TRH stimulation test – flat or absent response favours the diagnosis of hyperthyroidism (normal response – a rise in TSH to between 5–20 mU/l at 20 minutes, followed by a fall at 60 minutes)

Radiological Studies

Chest X-rays
    general screen for in-patients
    for out-patients indications are
        dyspnoea
        chest pain
        cyanosis
        congestive heart failure
        weight loss
        general ill-health
        confusion
        PUO
        osteomalacia to see Looser's zones
        signs in chest etc.
    (NB chest X-rays can be normal
        if lesion <6 mm in diameter
        in acute pulmonary embolism)

Skull X-rays
    indications
        trauma to detect fracture
        to see pineal and choroid plexus
        myeloma
        Paget's disease
        disseminated carcinoma

Plain abdomen indications
    suspected obstruction
    suspected perforation (erect and supine)
    renal colic
    cholecystitis
    chronic pancreatitis
    abdominal mass
    to see renal outlines in renal failure
    to confirm splenomegaly
    to assess constipation
    aortic aneurysm
    retroperitoneal haemorrhage

Barium swallow indications
    dysphagia
    signs and symptoms suggesting hiatus hernia
    to assess size of left atrium

Barium meal indications
    suspected peptic ulcer
    suspected gastric carcinoma
    investigation of anaemia
    investigation of upper abdominal mass
    haematemesis and melaena

Barium follow through – indicated in suspected
    coeliac disease
    Crohn's disease
    caecal carcinoma
    malabsorption

Barium enema
    indicated in patients with rectal bleeding in whom no lesion is
    seen on sigmoidoscopy
    suspected ischaemic colitis, pseudomembranous colitis, ul-
    cerative colitis, carcinoma or polyp

IVP (intravenous pyelogram)
    indications
        renal failure of unknown aetiology
        renal mass
        obstructive uropathy
    NB – high dose infusion pyleogram with tomography may be
    necessary if GFR is impaired

Cholecystogram used – used to demonstrate
    function of gall bladder
    presence of gall stones
    (not possible to do if serum bilirubin >30 mmol/l)

Intravenous cholangiogram
    usually done after cholecystectomy to see the state of biliary tree

Percutaneous transhepatic cholangiogram
    performed in patients with obstructive jaundice in whom other
    investigations including an isotopic scan have been unhelpful

Computerized transverse axial scanning of brain = computerized
    assisted tomography
    indications
        chronic subdural
        acute head trauma
        suspected brain atrophy

suspected cerebral tumour
normal pressure hydrocephalus
suspected abscess

Computerized tomography of whole body
useful in investigation of liver, pancreas, kidney, prostate and
bladder diseases

Radioisotope Investigations

Bone scanning
  isotopes used: $^{99}Tc^m$-labelled diphosphonate or pyrophosphate etc

  indications
    malignant bone disease
    osteomyelitis
    Paget's disease (especially in monitoring progress with treatment)
    bony pain (cause unknown)
    osteomalacia etc.
    abnormal bone biochemistry

Brain scanning
  isotopes available
    [$^{99}Tc^m$]pertechnetate

    [$^{99}Tc^m$]glucoheptonate

  indications
    suspected primary or secondary tumour
    chronic subdural (with dynamic studies)
    brain abscess
    cerebral infarction (in early stages it may be missed)
    (cf. transverse axial computerized scanning)

Cardiac imaging
  isotopes available
    thallium-201

    [$^{99}Tc^m$]pertechnetate etc.
  indications
    myocardial infarction
    diagnosis of ischaemic heart disease
    ventricular aneurysm
    left atrial myxoma

[^{125}I]fibrinogen uptake
  for suspected DVT in the leg
  high uptake confirms diagnosis

Liver scanning
  isotope used: $^{99}Tc^m$–sulphur colloid
  indications
    jaundice
    hepatomegaly

splenomegaly
to detect the presence of space occupying lesions prior to
biopsy
subphrenic abscess (combined lung–liver scanning)

for obstructive jaundice
[^{131}I]Rose Bengal (or ^{125}I-labelled)

[^{131}I]bromsulphthalein (or ^{125}I-labelled)
for suspected hepatoma or abscess use gallium-67

Lung scanning
isotopes used
for perfusion – ^{99}Tc^m-labelled microspheres or micro-
aggregates of albumin
for ventilation
krypton-81 or
xenon-133
indications
pulmonary embolism
subphrenic abscess

Pancreatic scanning – subtraction scan performed
isotopes used
[^{75}Se]selenomethionine

^{99}Tc^m-sulphur colloid
indications
pancreatic carcinoma
chronic pancreatitis
NB – high false +ve rate (20–30%)
investigations of choice in pancreatic disease are ERCP, ultrasound and X-ray computerized tomography

Renography
isotopes available
^{99}Tc^m-labelled diethylenetriamine
^{125}I-labelled hippuran
indications – obstructive uropathy – to assess the contribution of
each kidney to total function prior to and following surgery

Thyroid scanning
isotope used – [^{99}Tc^m]pertechnetate
indications
thyroid carcinoma
metastases from thyroid carcinoma

autonomous nodule
mediastinal extension of thyroid (for detection)

Ultrasound
   indications
      obstructive juandice
      pancreatic carcinoma
      chronic pancreatitis
      renal mass
      liver secondaries suspected in the left lobe
      thyroid swelling – to distinguish tumour from cyst
      to detect venous thrombosis

Electrocardiograph
   indications
      investigation of heart disease
      chest pain
      irregular pulse
      confusion
      cerebrovascular accident
      syncope
      falls (may need 24 hour monitoring to detect arrhythmias)
      dyspnoea
      hypotension
      hypothermia
      hyperkalaemia
      digoxin toxicity

Other Investigations

α-Fetoprotein
    high levels indicate hepatoma
    to a lesser extent high value can be found in viral hepatitis,
      cirrhosis and occasionally in GIT tumours with liver secon-
      daries
    (NB – negative result does not exclude hepatoma)

Cerebrospinal fluid
    lumbar puncture indicated in suspected
        meningitis ± encephalitis
        subarachnoid haemorrhage
        Guillain–Barré syndrome
        DS
        neurosyphilis
    (NB not indicated if SOL suspected)
    ↑protein found in
      meningitis
      encephalitis
      DS
      glioma, neurofibroma
      Guillain–Barré syndrome (very high)
      cord compression
    sugar
      absent or reduced in pyogenic meningitis
      reduced in
        tuberculous meningitis
        carcinomatous meningitis
    xanthochromia
      subarachnoid haemorrhage
      also found in
        intracerebral haemorrhage
        cerebral infarct
        obstruction of spinal subarachnoid space
    cells
      polymorphs
        pyogenic meningitis
        initially in viral meningitis
      mononuclear
        encephalitis, DS, polio, TB, herpes zoster
      mixed
        TB
        cerebral abscess

Cold agglutinins – present in
    mycoplasma pneumoniae infection
    lymphoma

Colonoscopy – indications
    for suspected colonic and rectal carcinoma
    rectal bleeding with negative X-rays
    biopsy of lesion seen on barium enema

Coomb's test – +ve in autoimmune haemolytic anaemia of aetiology
    idiopathic
    secondary to drugs (methyldopa)
    leukaemia
    lymphoma
    SLE
    rheumatoid arthritis
    myxoedema

Dexamethasone suppression test
    dexamethasone is a potent synthetic steroid which causes
        suppression of pituitary ACTH

    indications
        Cushing's syndrome – no suppression
        with high dose of dexamethasone there is suppression in
            Cushing's due to bilateral hyperplasia but not that due to
            adenoma or ectopic ACTH
        (NB – circadian rhythm absent in Cushing's)

Echocardiography
    examines the heart by reflected sound waves
    indications
        mitral valve disease
        left atrial myxoma
        prolapsing mitral valve
        pericardial effusion etc.

Electroencephalography
    records electrical activity of brain
    indicated in the diagnosis of epilepsy
    (NB – if history typical of epilepsy EEG not indicated)

Electromyography
    records electrical activity of muscles
    indication – muscle weakness of unknown aetiology

can distinguish muscle weakness due to neuropathy from that
due to primary muscle disease
characteristic changes in denervation, myasthenia, myotonia
etc.

Endoscopy
indications
dyspepsia with negative barium meal
haematemesis
for biopsy of lesion seen on barium meal
suspected oesophageal varices

ERCP (endoscopic retrograde cholangiopancreatography)
indicated in
suspected pancreatic disease – carcinoma as well as
chronic pancreatitis
biliary disease where other investigations have been
equivocal

Faecal fat excretion
5-day complete collection necessary
normal value <18 mmol/24 hours
indication: suspected steatorrhoea
NB – other tests of malabsorption are
xylose excretion test (oral and i.v.)
barium follow through
jejunal biopsy indicated in suspected
coeliac disease,
lymphoma
Whipple's disease
^{14}C breath test for suspected blind loop syndrome

Ham's test
+ve acidified serum lysis test
+ve in paroxysmal nocturnal haemoglobulinuria

Kveim test
intracutaneous injection of human sarcoid tissue
+ve in sarcoidosis in 50–80% of patients
false positive result may be obtained in patients with other
granulomatous conditions or collagen vascular diseases

Laparoscopy
carried out under local or general anaesthetic

for examination and biopsy of abdominal organs: liver, pancreas, peritoneum etc.

LE cell
    presence suggests SLE
    but can also be found in
        rheumatoid arthritis
        patients taking practolol, procainamide etc.
    presence of anti-DNA antibodies and extractable nuclear antigen (ENA) favours diagnosis of SLE

Liver biopsy
    indications
        biopsy of space occupying lesion seen on scan
        diagnosis of suspected liver disease when other tests including a scan have been negative
        monitor result of treatment of chronic active hepatitis

Mediastinoscopy
    for diagnosis and biopsy of tumour or cyst in mediastinum e.g. lymphoma, bronchogenic carcinoma etc.

Mitochondrial antibody test
    +ve in primary biliary cirrhosis
    +ve in minority of patients with cirrhosis, obstructive jaundice and chronic active hepatitis

Muscle biopsy
    indications
        to differentiate myopathy from neuromyopathy
        for suspected diagnosis of
            polymyositis
            polyarteritis nodosa etc.

Nerve conduction studies
    indication – suspected peripheral neuropathy

Pleural fluid
    aspiration indicated
        where aetiology of effusion not clinically clear
        for symptomatic relief

    high protein indicates exudate (infection, malignancy etc.)
    low protein indicates transudate (congestive heart failure, cirrhosis, low serum albumin)
    low sugar – rheumatoid arthritis

high amylase – pancreatitis
cells
>neutrophils – suggest bacterial infection
>lymphocytes – suggest tuberculosis
>giant multinucleated cells – suggest rheumatoid arthritis
>malignant cells – suggest involvement of pleura by tumour
>>(if malignant effusion suspected pleural biopsy should
>>be taken at the time of aspiration)

Precipitating antibodies – detected in
pulmonary aspergillosis
Micropolyspora spp. (Farmer's lung)

Respiratory function tests
>obstructive airways diseases (asthma, emphysema etc.) have
>>$FEV_1\downarrow$, $PEFR\downarrow$, $FEV_1/FVC\downarrow$
>restrictive airways diseases have low FEV_1 and FVC but the ratio
>>is normal, i.e. over 75%
>cf. respiratory failure see p. 169

Rose–Waller test
+ve in rheumatoid arthritis
can also be +ve in
>SLE
>chronic infection
>cirrhosis
>fibrosing alveolitis
negative in
>gout
>Reiter's syndrome
>ankylosing spondylitis
>arthritis associated with
>>psoriasis
>>ulcerative colitis

Serological tests – for suspected
brucellosis
Mycoplasma pneumoniae infection
rickettsia infection
psittacosis
viruses
>adenoviruses, influenza A, B and C etc.
>need a pair of sera to show significant rise of antibodies
>>during course of illness

NB – viruses can be isolated from infected specimen and grown as well as seen under microscope
light microscope: herpes inclusion bodies
electron – pox viruses etc.

Synacthen (tetracosactrin) test
synacthen is a biologically active part of ACTH which stimulates adrenal cortex
normal response
rise in serum cortisol of at least 200 nmol/l to at least 800 nmol/l after 250 µg of tetracosactrin

subnormal response
obtained in primary adrenal insufficiency in which ACTH is high
subnormal or delayed response
obtained in secondary adrenal insufficiency in which serum ACTH is low

Uric acid
raised in gout, although often it is found to be normal – diagnosis of gout made on clinical signs and symptoms ± finding of crystals (negatively refractile) of monosodium urate
↑renal failure
in myeloproliferative diseases and other conditions in which cell turnover is high

Urine and plasma osmolality
indications
to distinguish dehydration from acute tubular necrosis
to diagnose inappropriate ADH secretion

ratio of urine:plasma osmolality >2 suggests prerenal failure

ratio of urine:plasma osmolality <1.7 suggests ATN

reduced plasma osmolality with urine osmolality >300 mosm/l indicates inappropriate ADH secretion

Normal Values

Blood

acid phosphatase	up to 0.7 U/l
albumin	32.9–49.3 g/l
alkaline phosphatase	21–93 U/l
amylase	70–300 U/l
bicarbonate	19.5–30.7 mmol/l
bilirubin (total)	2–14 μmol/l
calcium (total)	2.1–2.59 mmol/l (men)
	2.18–2.68 mmol/l (women)
cholesterol	4.1–8.9 mmol/l (men)
	4.7–11.2 mmol/l (women)
cortisol (10 a.m.)	280–720 nmol/l
creatinine	52–169 μmol/l
creatine phosphokinase	up to 60 U/l
HBD (hydroxybutyrate dehydrogenase)	70–190 U/l
iron	10–28 μmol/l (women)
	14–32 μmol/l (men)
iron binding capacity	up to 71 $u$mol/l
magnesium	0.7–1.0 mmol/l
osmolarity	260–309 mosm/l
PCO_2	4.6–6.0 kPa
phosphate	0.67–1.31 mmol/l (men)
	0.71–31 mmol/l (women)
PO_2	9.3–13.3 kPa
potassium	3.5–5.2 mmol/l
red cell folate	160–640 ng/ml
serum B_{12}	100–1000 pg/ml
serum folate	6–21 ng/ml
SGOT (asparate transaminase)	9–27 U/l (men)
	8–24 U/l (women)
sodium	132–142 mmol/l
thyrotropin (TSH)	less than 4 mU/l
thyroxine	57–129 nmol/l
tri-iodothyronine (T_3)	1.0–0.28 nmol/l
urea	3.9–9.9 mmol/l
uric acid	180–470 mmol/l (men)
	120–460 mmol/l (women)
zinc	12–23 μmol/l

Urine

calcium	5–10 mmol/24 h
5HIAA (5-hydroxyindole acetic acid)	trace
magnesium	0.2–12 mmol/24 h
osmolarity	Over 300 mmol/l
phosphorus	22–32 mmol/24 h
protein	nil
uric acid	3–12 mmol/24 h
potassium	20–60 mmol/24 h
protein	nil
sodium	50–200 mmol/24 h
urea	330–500 mmol/24 h
uric acid	3–12 mmol/24 h

Faeces

fat	<18 mmol/24 h

CSF

glucose	2.5–5.3 mmol/l
pressure	70–200 mm of water
protein (lumbar)	0.1–0.4 g/l

(NB normal values may vary a little from lab to lab)

Index